ELECTROCARDIOGRAPHY

ELECTROCARDIOGRAPHY

A GUIDE FOR PHYSICIANS, MEDICAL
STUDENTS, NURSE PRACTITIONERS,
AND OTHER
HEALTHCARE PROVIDERS

H. THOMAS MILHORN, MD, PHD

Universal-Publishers
Irvine • Boca Raton

Electrocardiography: A Guide for Physicians, Medical Students,
Nurse Practitioners, and Other Healthcare Providers

Universal Publishers, Inc.
Irvine, California & Boca Raton, Florida • USA
www.Universal-Publishers.com
2018

ISBN: 978-1-62734-259-9 (pbk.)
ISBN: 978-1-62734-260-5 (ebk.)

Typeset by Medlar Publishing Solutions Pvt Ltd, India

Cover design by Ivan Popov

Publisher's Cataloging-in-Publication Data

Names: Milhorn, H. Thomas, author.
Title: Electrocardiography : a guide for physicians, medical students,
    nurse practitioners, and other healthcare providers / H. Thomas
    Milhorn.
Description: Irvine, CA : Universal Publishers, 2018.
Identifiers: LCCN 2018952193 | ISBN 978-1-62734-259-9 (pbk.) |
    ISBN 978-1-62734-260-5 (ebook)
Subjects: LCSH: Electrocardiography. | Heart--Diseases--Diagnosis.
    | Chest pain. | Myocardial infarction--Diagnosis. | Syncope (Pathology) | Sudden death. | BISAC: MEDICAL / Cardiology. | MEDICAL / Diagnosis.
Classification: LCC RC683.5.E5 M55 (print) | LCC RC683.5.E5
    (ebook) | DDC 616.1/207547--dc23.

PREFACE

The electrocardiogram can serve as an independent identifier of myocardial disease or reflect anatomic, metabolic, hemodynamic, or electrophysiological alterations in the heart. It can provide information that is often essential for the proper diagnosis and treatment of a variety of disorders and is without equal as a method for diagnosing cardiac arrhythmias. It is the procedure of choice for patients who present with chest pain, dizziness, syncope, or symptoms that may indicate risk of myocardial infarction or sudden death.

Primary care physicians are often the first, and sometimes the only, point of contact for many patients within the health care system. The standard 12-lead electrocardiogram is one of the most common tests obtained and interpreted by the primary care physician, with most physicians reading their own recordings and basing clinical decisions on their findings. It has been shown that primary care physicians can achieve proficiency in the interpretation of over 95 percent of all electrocardiogram findings seen in the primary care setting.

Although computerized interpretation is widely available, it is considered unreliable in up to 20 percent of the cases, making interpretation by primary care physicians an essential skill. This book provides the necessary skills for primary care physicians to use in interpreting electrocardiograms, both in their offices and in the emergency departments of their hospitals.

As the subtitle states, this book is about the essential elements involved in electrocardiographic interpretation. It is not all inclusive; however, it does cover the abnormalities most likely to be seen by primary care physicians in their everyday practice of medicine.

This book is the result of a course I taught in the Department of Family Medicine at the University of Mississippi School of Medicine and five articles titled *Electrocardiography for the*

Family Physician I subsequently published in *Family Practice Recertification.*

In short, this book is the one I wish I had access to during the many years I actively practiced family medicine and when I was a resident in family medicine.

Although this book was written with the primary care physician in mind, it should prove useful to medical students, residents in all primary care specialties, primary care nurse practitioners, and physician assistants. It is an outgrowth of my prior book *Electrocardiography for the Family Physician.*

I currently teach an electrocardiography course to family medicine residents in the EC-Healthnet Family Medicine Residency Program in Meridian, Mississippi.

H. Thomas Milhorn, MD, PhD
www.milhornbooks.net

Contents

Chapter 1

The Electrocardiogram

Electrocardiography is a test that measures the electrical signals that control the rhythm of the heartbeat. The graph that shows the results is called an *electrocardiogram* (EKG, ECG).

An electrocardiogram may show:

- Abnormal conduction of cardiac impulses due to damage of the conducting system
- Abnormally slow, fast, or irregular heart rhythms
- Adverse effects on the heart from certain lung conditions, such as emphysema and pulmonary embolus
- Adverse effects on the heart from various cardiovascular or systemic diseases, such as high blood pressure and thyroid conditions
- Certain congenital heart abnormalities
- Changes in the electrical activity of the heart caused by medication (digoxin, type 1a antiarrhythmics such as quinidine)
- Evidence of abnormal blood electrolytes (potassium, calcium)
- Evidence of an acute impairment of blood flow to the heart (angina)
- Evidence of an acute, evolving, or prior myocardial infarction
- Evidence of atrial enlargement or ventricular hypertrophy
- Evidence of inflammation of the heart (myocarditis) or its lining (pericarditis).

ELECTROCARDIOGRAPH PAPER

The electrocardiogram is recorded on graph paper with divisions as indicated in Figure 1-1. Since the ECG paper speed is ordinarily 25 mm/second, a small square is 0.04 seconds wide. A small square is one millimeter (0.1 mV) high. A large square is 0.2 seconds wide and five millimeters (0.5 mV) high.

A square-wave *calibration signal* is placed on every electrocardiogram. When recorded with a normal calibration, the signal is 10 mm high and represents 1.0 mV. When recorded at half standard, because of large QRS voltages, the calibration standard is 5 millimeters, also representing 1.0 mV. The calibration standard should always be noted first when interpreting an electrocardiogram. The full-standard calibration is used throughout this book.

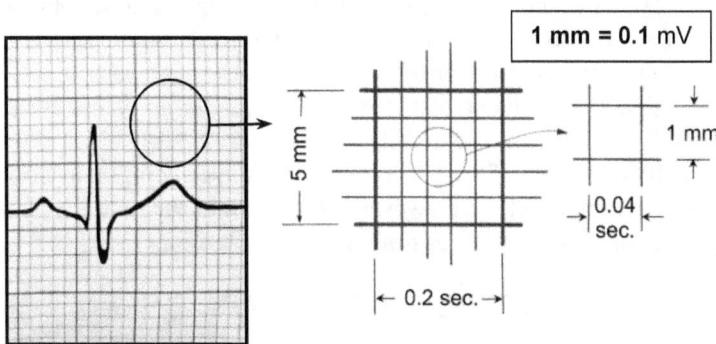

Figure 1-1. Electrocardiograph paper dimensions (full standard).

CONDUCTION SYSTEM OF THE HEART

Electrical activation of the atrial and ventricular muscle is termed *depolarization*. Initiation of depolarization normally occurs in the *sinoatrial node (SA node)*. The current then travels through the *internodal tracts* of the atria to the *atrioventricular node (AV node)*. From there the depolarization wave passes down the *bundle of His (atrioventriclular bundle)*, which divides into the *right* and *left bundle branches* (Figure 1-2).

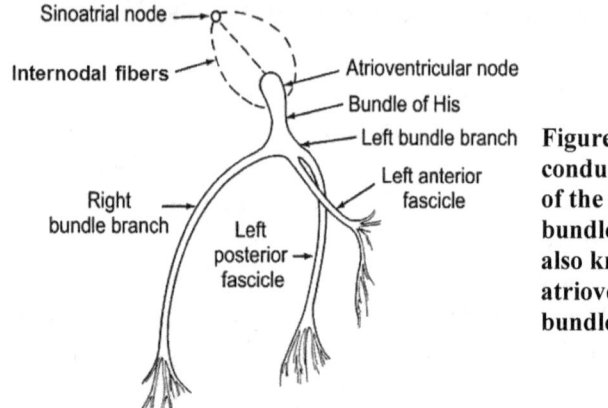

Figure 1-2. The conduction system of the heart. The bundle of His is also known as the atrioventricular bundle

The left bundle branch, in turn, divides into the *left anterior* and *left posterior fascicles*. The right bundle branch is not divided and supplies the right ventricle. The left bundle branch supplies the left ventricle. The AV node, bundle of His, and right and left bundle branches are known collectively as the *Purkinje* system. The depolarization wave rapidly spreads out from these pathways, causing contraction of the myocardial muscle. *Repolarization* of the electrical potential of the cardiac muscle cells follows.

The blood supply of the SA and AV nodes usually originates from the right coronary artery. However, ten percent of the time the blood supply to the AV node arises from the circumflex artery.

PARTS OF THE ELECTROCARDIOGRAM

Because the body is a conductor of electrical current, the electrical activity of the heart can be monitored by the use of a galvanometer and electrodes placed on the surface of the skin. Depolarization and repolarization result in various deflections recorded on ECG paper. From this recording, various waves, intervals, and segments can be identified.

Deflections

The *P wave* reflects atrial depolarization, the *QRS complex* reflects ventricular depolarization, and the *T wave* reflects ventricular repolarization (Figure 1-3). Atrial repolarization occurs during

3

ventricular depolarization and, therefore, is obscured by the QRS complex.

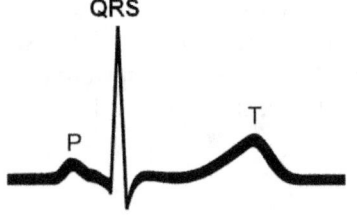

Figure 1-3. The deflections of the electrocardiogram generated by the heart during depolarization and repolarization.

P Wave

The *P wave* is normally largest in lead II and positive in leads I, II and V_3-V_6. It is normally negative in lead aV_R and may be biphasic in leads V_1 and V_2. If the P wave is not upright in lead II, you should suspect:

- Dextrocardia
- Ectopic atrial rhythm
- Reversed arm electrodes

The P wave normally lasts less than 0.11 seconds (just less than three small squares). An abnormally long P wave occurs whenever it takes extra time for the electrical wave to travel over the entire atrium, such as in atrial enlargement. The height of the P wave is normally less than 2.5 small squares (0.25 mV).

An abnormally tall P wave is seen when larger amounts of electricity are moving over the atrium than normally, such as also occurs in atrial enlargement. Abnormal P waves can be:

- **Widened.** Treatment with a Class Ia antiarrhythmic agent, such as quinidine
- **Inverted.** Direction opposite the predominant QRS deflection. Retrograde atrial depolarization; that is, depolarization originating low in the atria or in the atrioventricular junction and traveling backward up the atria
- **Notched.** Atrial enlargement
- **Small or Absent.** Hyperkalemia

4

QRS Complex

The *QRS complex* represents depolarization of the ventricles. By definition, the *Q wave* is the first downward stroke of the QRS complex and is usually followed by an *R wave*, which is the first upward deflection of the QRS complex. An *S wave* is an upward deflection that is preceded by a downward deflection (Figure 1-4).

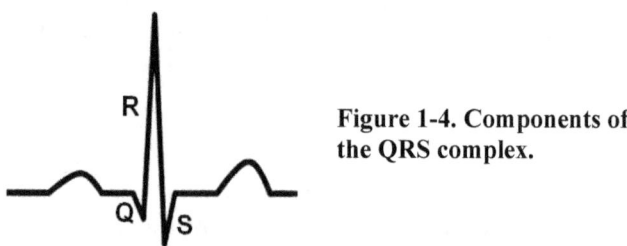

Figure 1-4. Components of the QRS complex.

A QRS complex may not necessarily contain a Q wave, an R wave, or an S wave, and may contain more than one R wave (Figure 1-5).

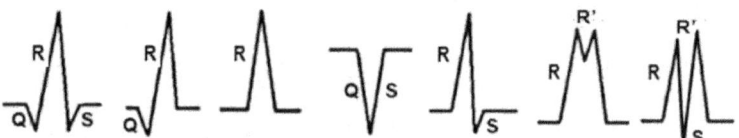

Figure 1-5. Examples of various QRS complex morphologies and their nomenclatures

If a second upward deflection is seen, it is called an R-prime (R') wave. An R followed by an extension below the baseline is an S, giving an RSR'. RR' and RSR' waves are never normal in adults but indicate a problem in the ventricular conduction system.

Causes of an RR' or RSR' include bundle branch block and incomplete bundle branch block. An RSR' configuration can be normal in the right-most chest lead (V₁) of young children.

The width of the QRS complex is the time required for the ventricular cells to depolarize. The normal duration is 0.06 to 0.10 seconds (1-1/2 to 2-1/2 small squares).

Lengthening of the QRS interval usually indicates some blockage of the electrical activity in the conducting system. Some causes of increased QRS duration include:

- Drug effect (procainamide, tricyclic antidepressants, cocaine)
- Electrolyte effect (hyperkalemia, hypermagnesemia)
- Premature ventricular contractions
- Right and left bundle branch blocks
- Supraventricular beats with aberration
- Ventricular escape beats
- Ventricular pacemaker beats
- Wolff-Parkinson-White syndrome

T Wave

The *T wave* represents the wave of repolarization as the ventricle muscle prepares for firing again. It is normally upright in all leads except aV_R and V_1. It is normally inverted in lead aV_R.

The height of the T wave is normally less than five millimeters (0.5 mV) in the standard limb leads and less than 10 mm (1.0 mV) in the precordial leads. The direction normally follows the direction of the main QRS deflection. T wave abnormalities may be seen with or without ST segment abnormalities. T wave abnormalities include:

- **Tall T waves.** Hyperkalemia, very early myocardial infarction, and left ventricular hypertrophy
- **Flat or small T waves.** Ischemia, evolving myocardial infarction, myocarditis, pulmonary embolus, hypokalemia, thick chest wall, emphysema, pericardial effusion, cardiomyopathy, constrictive pericarditis, hypothyroidism, hypoadrenalism, hypocalcemia, and nonspecific causes
- **Inverted T waves.** Ischemia, infarction, late in pericarditis, left ventricular hypertrophy, bundle branch blocks, digoxin, athletic heart syndrome, and acute cerebral disease

In young children, T waves normally may be inverted in the right precordial leads (V_1 to V_3). Occasionally, these T wave inversions persist into young adulthood.

Concordance and discordance

Concordance and discordance have to do with the direction of the T wave in relation to the direction of the QRS complex).

- **Concordance**: The direction of the T wave is in the same direction as that of the main QRS deflection (Figure 1-6A)
- **Discordance:** The direction of the T wave is in the opposite direction than that of the main QRS deflection (Figure 1-6B)

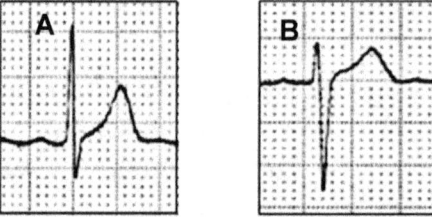

Figure 1-6. (A) Concordance and (B) discordance.

U Wave

When present, a second wave following the T wave is called a *U wave* (Figure 1-7). Its direction usually is the same as that of the T wave. Its amplitude is usually less than 1/3 of the T wave amplitude in the same lead.

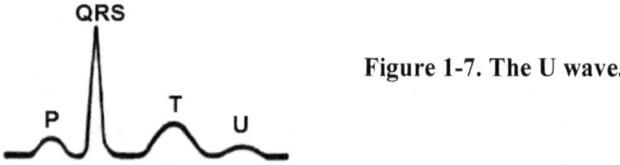

Figure 1-7. The U wave.

U waves are most prominent in leads V_2 and V_3. Their Usual direction is the same as the T wave; however, in some cases they may be inverted.

The most common cause of prominent U waves is bradycardia, generally becoming visible when the heart rate falls below 65 bpm. Other causes of positive U waves are:

- CNS disease
- Drugs (amiodarone, disopyramide, digoxin, epinephrine, phenothiazines, procainamide , quinidine)
- Electrolyte imbalance (hypokalemia, hypomagnesemia, hypercalcemia)
- Hyperthyroidism
- Left ventricular hypertrophy
- Long QT syndrome
- Mitral valve prolapse

Inverted U waves may be seen with:

- Coronary artery spasm (Prinzmetal's angina)
- Myocardial infarction
- During episode of acute ischemia
- Some cases of left ventricular hypertrophy or right ventricular hypertrophy
- Some patients with long QT syndrome

The exact significance of U waves is unknown, but they may be due to repolarization of the papillary muscles or Purkinje fibers.

Intervals

The PR, QRS, and QT intervals fall within well-defined limits (Figure 1-8).

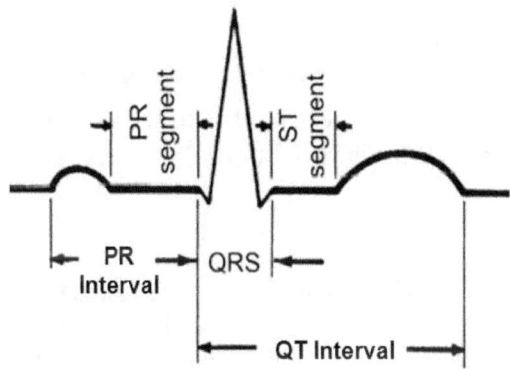

Figure 1-8. Intervals and segments in the electrocardiogram.

PR Interval

The *PR interval* is the time required for the depolarization wave to complete atrial depolarization; be conducted through the AV node, bundle of His and bundle branches; and arrive at the ventricular myocardial cells. It is the time from the beginning of the P wave to the beginning of the QRS complex. It is normally between 0.12 and 0.2 seconds (three to five small squares) in length.

The PR interval may be prolonged when conduction of the electrical wave through the AV node is slow. This may be seen with:

- Degenerative disease of the AV node
- Digoxin, beta blockers, some calcium channel blockers (diltiazem, verapamil)
- Electrolyte abnormalities (hyperkalemia, hypercalcemia)
- Hypothermia
- Hyperthyroidism

The PR interval may be unusually short with:

- Electrolyte abnormalities (hypokalemia, hypocalcemia)
- Hypertrophic cardiomyopathy
- Type II glycogen storage disease (Pompe's disease)
- Junctional rhythm
- Pacing
- Hypertension
- Tachycardia
- Preexcitation syndromes (Wolff-Parkinson-White syndrome, Lown-Ganong-Levine syndrome)

QT Interval

The *QT interval* is the time required for depolarization and repolarization of the ventricles, measured from the beginning of the QRS complex to the end of the T wave. The normal QT interval varies with heart rate. Fast rates shorten the QT interval and slow heart rates lengthen it.

At normal heart rates the QT interval lasts between 0.34 and 0.42 seconds. A way to compensate for changes in the QT interval with heart rate is to use a formula such as Hodge's formula:

$$QTc = QT + 0.00175(heart\ rate - 60)$$

where QTc is the corrected QT interval. The formula corrects QT for all ECGs to a heart rate of 60 bpm.

The corrected QT interval (QTc) should be less than 0.44 seconds in males and 0.46 seconds in females. If the QTc is prolonged there is a risk of ventricular arrhythmia, in particular Torsades de pointes. Torsades de pointes is a ventricular tachycardia characterized by fluctuation of the QRS complex magnitudes around the electrocardiographic baseline (Figure 1-9).

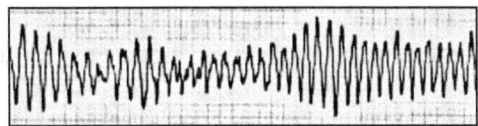

Figure 1-9. Torsades de pointes

Females normally have a QT interval slightly longer than that of males.

The QT interval may be prolonged with:

- Over 50 medications, including amiodarone, chlorpromazine, clarithromycin, erythromycin, haloperidol, thioridazine, type Ia antiarrhythmic agents (quinidine, procainamide, disopyramide), and other antiarrhythmics.
- Congestive heart failure
- Hypothyroidism
- Hypothermia
- Electrolyte abnormalities (hypokalemia, hypocalcemia, hypomagnesemia)
- Myocardial ischemia and infarction
- Myocarditis
- Organophosphate insecticide poisoning
- Severe CNS events (seizures, CVA, intracranial hemorrhage)
- Hereditary diseases (Jervell and Lang Nielson syndrome, Romano Ward syndrome)

Other formulas for calculating QTc are:

- Linear formula
  - Framingham formula: $QTc = QT + 0.154 (1 - RR)$
- Logarithmic formulas
  - Bazett's formula: $QTc = QT/(RR)^{0.5}$
  - Fridericia's formula: $QTc = QT/(RR)^{0.33}$
  - Baseline correction: $QTc = QT/(RR)^{0.37}$

All formulas give similar results.

Segments

PR Segment

The *PR segment* is the portion of the tracing falling between the end of the P wave and the beginning of the QRS complex. During this time, the electrical wave moves slowly through the atrioventricular node. The PR segment is not routinely measured but may be commented on if it is depressed or elevated. A common cause of PR segment depression is pericarditis.

ST Segment

The *ST segment* is the portion of the tracing falling between the end of the QRS complex and the beginning of the T wave. During this time, the ventricle is contracting, but no electricity is flowing. The ST segment is therefore usually at the baseline. ST segment elevation or depression is generally measured at a point two small squares beyond the end of the QRS complex.

The length of the ST segment shortens with increasing heart rate. Measurement of the length of the ST segment alone is usually not of any clinical use; however, ST segment depression and elevation can be clinically important.

ST segment depression can occur with:

- Acute posterior myocardial infarction
- Angina

- Drug effects (digoxin, quinidine)
- Electrolyte effects (hypokalemia, hypercalcemia, hypermagnesium)
- Hypothermia
- Left bundle branch block
- Pulmonary embolus
- Reciprocal changes representing cardiac injury in other leads
- Supraventricular tachycardia
- Ventricular hypertrophy with strain

ST segment elevation can occur with:

- Acute pericarditis
- Myocarditis
- Athletic heart syndrome
- Brugada syndrome (congenital abnormality)
- Cardiomyopathy
- CNS events, such as subarachnoid hemorrhage
- Early repolarization
- Hyperkalemia
- Left ventricular aneurysm
- Reciprocal changes due to ischemia in other leads
- ST-segment elevation myocardial infarction
- Vasospasm (Prinzmetal's angina, cocaine or methamphetamine abuse)

ST-T Complex

The *repolarization complex* (ST-T) is the most sensitive part of the electrocardiogram. It consists of the ST segment and the T wave. ST-T complexes can change in duration, amplitude, and sign, or combinations of these. The ST-T complex can be influenced by many nonpathological factors, including temperature, hyperventilation, and anxiety.

The diagnosis of *nonspecific ST-T abnormality* is made when the repolarization complex is abnormal, but not suggestive of a specific diagnosis. The most common nonspecific ST-T abnormality is low T wave voltages with slight sagging or flattening of the ST segment (Figure 1-10).

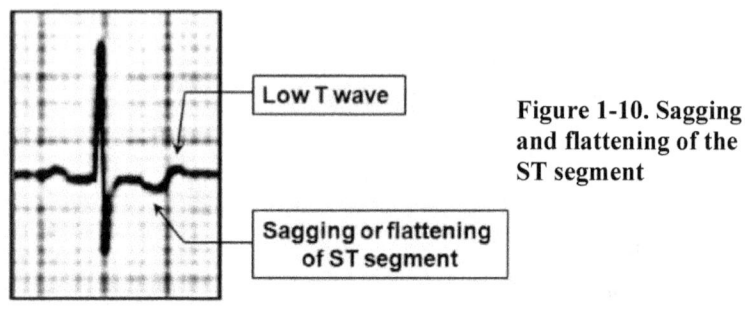

Low T wave

Sagging or flattening
of ST segment

Figure 1-10. Sagging and flattening of the ST segment

J Point

The *J point* marks the end of ventricular depolarization (Figure 1-11). It is the point of intersection between the end of the QRS complex and the onset of the ST segment. As such, it is an essential landmark for measuring QRS duration. At times, the J point can be difficult to identify.

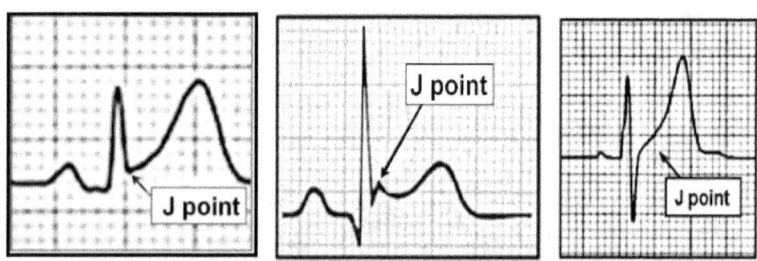

J point

J point

J point

Figure 1-11. The J Point.

ELECTROCARDIOGRAPHIC INTERPRETATION

In interpreting an ECG, one looks in order at eight areas on each ECG:

1. Calibration standard (half or full standard)
2. Rate (normal, greater than normal, less than normal)
3. Rhythm (regular, regularly irregular, irregularly irregular)
4. Axis (normal axis, left axis deviation, right axis deviation, etc.)
5. Intervals (PR, QRS, QT), segments (PR, ST)
6. Signs of atrial enlargement or ventricular hypertrophy (P wave morphology, greater than normal magnitudes of QRS complexes)
7. Signs of ischemia and infarction (ST segment elevations and depressions, Q waves)
8. Other findings

If there is a previous ECG in the patient's file, the current ECG should be compared with it to see if any significant changes have occurred.

From all of the above information, taking into account the patient's symptoms and history, we arrive at an ECG interpretation.

Chapter 1 Quiz

Electrocardiograph paper (questions 1 to 4)

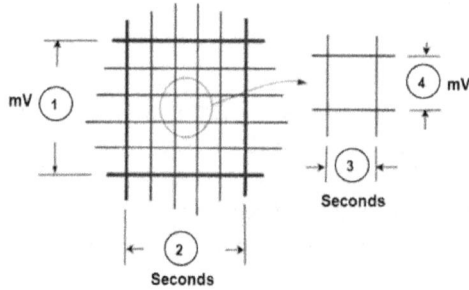

5. PR interval
6. QT interval
7. QRS width
8. PR segment
9. ST segment

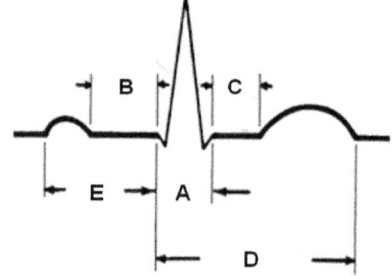

10. What is the magnitude of the J-point in mV)?

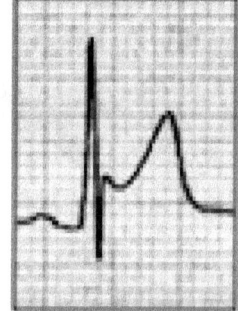

11. RR'
12. QS
13. QR
14. RS
15. R
16. QRS
17. RSR'

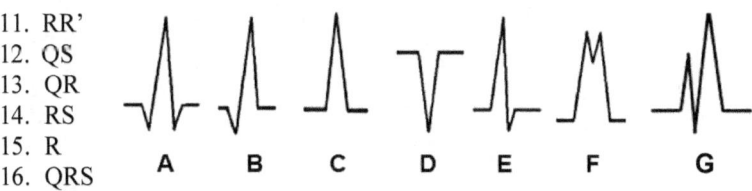

A   B   C   D   E   F   G

18. If the heart rate is 120 bpm and QT is 0.44 seconds, what is the corrected QT (QTc) using Hodge's formula?

19. Is the corrected QT (QTc) above:
    A. Normal
    B. Prolonged
    C. Short
    D. Both prolonged and short (Schrödinger's QTc)

Chapter 2

Leads and the Normal Electrocardiogram

LEADS

Two types of arrangements of leads are used—bipolar leads and unipolar leads.

Bipolar Leads

A *bipolar lead* is one in which the electrical activity at one electrode is compared with that of another electrode, the net result being the measurement of electrical activity between the two electrodes (Figure 2-1).

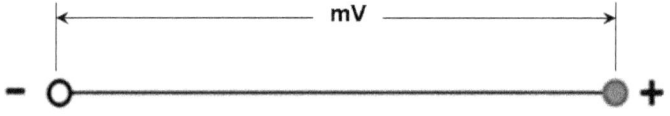

Figure 2-1. Formation of a bipolar lead.

By convention, a positive electrode is one in which the electrocardiograph records a positive (upward) signal when the electrical impulse flows toward it and a negative (downward) signal when the electrical impulse flows away from it.

Figure 2-2 shows depolarization of a hypothetical strip of cardiac muscle and the corresponding generation of the electrocardiogram tracing. In segment A the muscle is in its normal state of polarization. Hence, the electrocardiogram recorded from both ends is at zero. In segment B the depolarization wave is traveling away from the electrode at the left and toward the one at the right. This results in a negative deflection in the left electrode and a positive deflection in the right electrode. In segment C the muscle strip is completely depolarized so the electrocardiogram tracings have returned to zero.

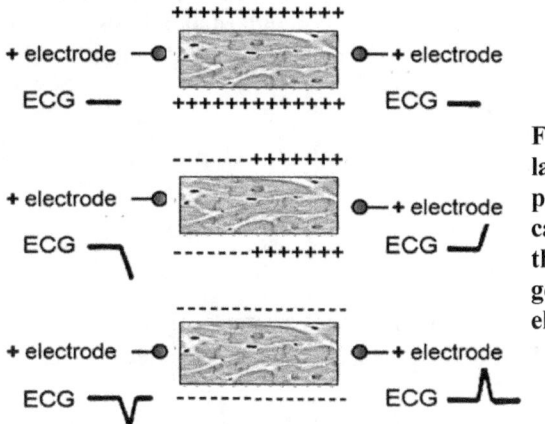

Figure 2-2. Depolarization of a hypothetical strip of cardiac muscle and the corresponding generation of the electrocardiogram.

Standard Limb Leads

By attaching electrodes to the left arm, right arm, and left leg, we obtain the three bipolar *standard limb leads*, named I, II, and III.

The standard limb lead placements are formed as follows:

- **Lead I:** Negative electrode placed on the right arm and positive electrode placed on the left arm
- **Lead II:** Negative electrode placed on the right arm and positive electrode placed on the left leg
- **Lead III:** Negative electrode placed on the left arm and positive electrode placed on the left leg

The three standard limb leads form an imaginary triangle (Einthoven's triangle) having the heart at its "center" and formed by lines that represent the three standard limb leads of the electrocardiogram. Placement of the standard limb leads are shown in Figure 2-3.

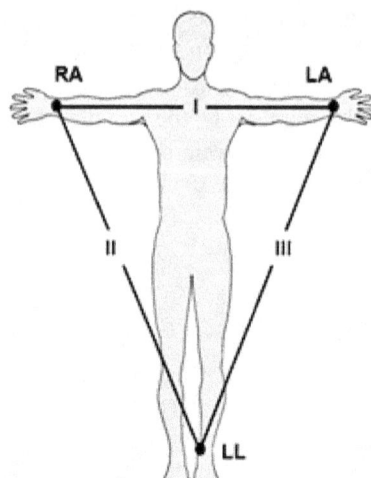

Figure 2-3. Placement of the standard limb leads to form Einthoven's triangle.

The right arm and left arm electrodes alternatively may be placed on the right and left shoulders, respectively. The leg electrode can be placed on the thigh.

The standard limb leads explore the electrical activity of the heart in a frontal plane; that is, the orientation of the heart seen when looking directly at the anterior chest (Figure 2-4).

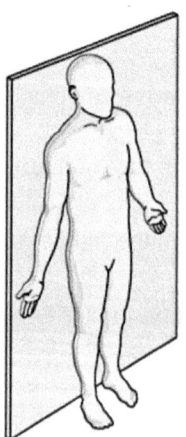

Figure 2-4. The frontal plane.

The standard limb leads form a set of axes 60 degrees apart (Figure 2-5).

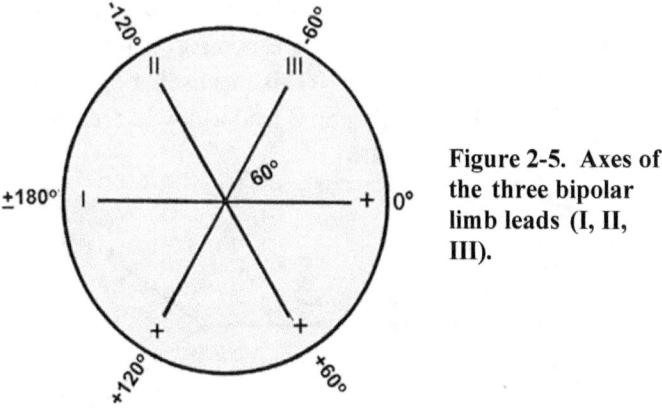

Figure 2-5. Axes of the three bipolar limb leads (I, II, III).

Unipolar Leads

A *unipolar lead* is one in which the electrical potential at an electrode is compared to a reference point that averages electrical activity of combined leads. The single electrode, termed the *exploring electrode*, is the positive electrode.

There are two sets of unipolar leads—the augmented limb leads and the chest (precordial) leads.

Augmented Limb Leads

A second set of limb leads (aV$_R$, aV$_L$, AV$_F$) are unipolar leads. The "a" stands augmented, "V" for voltage, "R" for right arm, "L" for left arm, and "F" for foot. They are referred to as augmented leads because an electrical manipulation is done to increase the size of the voltage recordings.

In actuality, augmented limb leads use the same electrodes as leads I, II, and III. The ECG machine switches and rearranges the electrode designations.

Each augmented lead is formed by combining the potentials from two electrodes to form the exploring electrode, which becomes the positive electrode.

The augmented leads are formed as follows:

- **Lead aV$_R$:** Created by connecting the left arm and the foot (leg) electrodes together to form the negative "electrode." The voltage of this average electrode is compared to the right arm electrode (positive electrode). This means that if electricity is moving in a rightward direction, lead aV$_R$ will record an upward deflection (Figure 2-6).

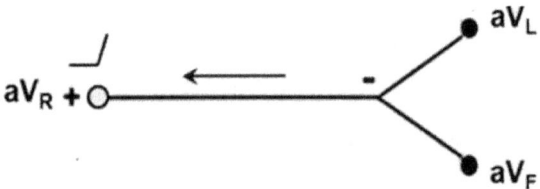

Figure 2-6. Formation of the augmented lead aV$_R$.

- **Lead aV$_L$:** Created by connecting the right arm and the foot together to form a negative "electrode," then comparing this "average" electrode to the left arm electrode. The left arm electrode is positive, meaning that electricity moving to the left will cause an upward deflection in lead aV$_L$ (Figure 2-7).

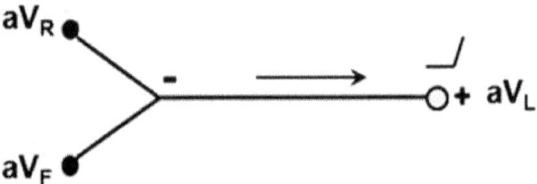

Figure 2-7. Formation of the augmented lead aV$_L$.

- **Lead aV$_F$:** Created by connecting the two arm leads together to create an "average" electrode. To the ECG machine, this combination looks like a single negative electrode midway between the two arms (directly in the center of the body above the heart). This "average" electrode is connected through the ECG machine to the foot electrode. The foot is the positive electrode, so a downward motion of electricity will make the ECG stylus move upward on the paper in a lead V$_F$ (Figure 2-8).

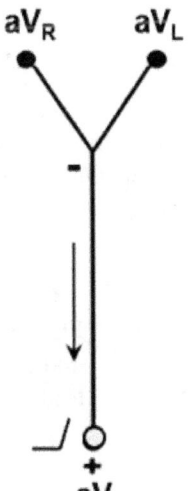

Figure 2-8. Formation of the augmented lead aV$_F$.

Combined standard and Augmented Limb Leads

The augmented limb leads, like the standard limb leads, form a set of axes 60 degrees apart. However, the axes of the augmented limb leads are rotated 30 degrees from the axes of the standard limb leads. This very conveniently gives a lead every 30 degrees. (Figure 2-9).

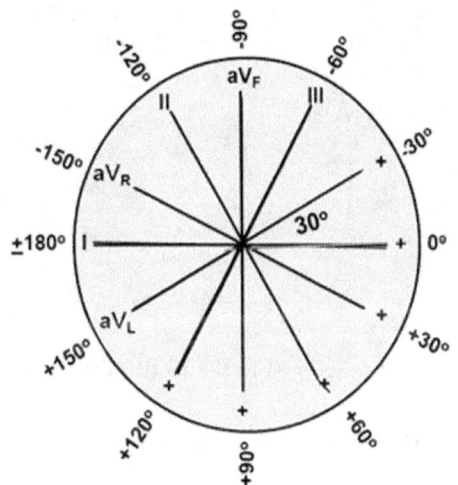

Figure 2-9. Axes of all six limb leads (I, II, III, aV$_L$, aV$_R$, aV$_F$).

Chest Leads

The six *chest (precordial) leads* (V_1, V_2, V_3, V_4, V_5, V_6) are unipolar leads that explore the electrical activity of the heart in a horizontal plane. The reference point is obtained by connecting the left arm, right arm, and left leg electrodes together (Figure 2-10). The positive electrode is the exploring electrode.

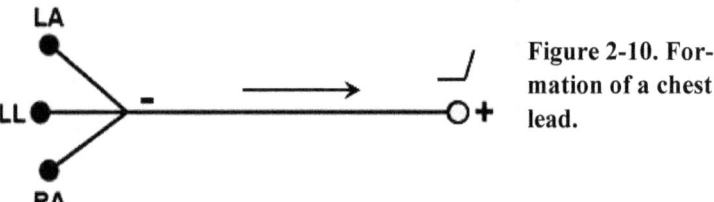

Figure 2-10. Formation of a chest lead.

The standard positions for the exploring chest electrodes are located with reference to various landmarks of the bony thorax (Figure 2-11).

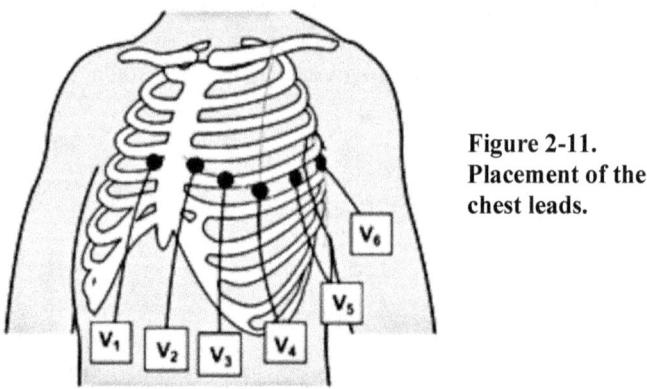

Figure 2-11. Placement of the chest leads.

Their locations are:

- V_1 is in the fourth intercostal space just to the right of the sternum.
- V_2 is at the fourth intercostal space just to the left of the sternum.

- V_3 is halfway between V_2 and V_4.
- V_4 is at the fifth intercostal space in the midclavicular line.
- V_5 is in the anterior axillary line at the same level as V_4.
- V_6 is at the same level in the midaxillary line.

The chest leads explore the electrical activity of the heart in a horizontal (transverse) plane; that is, as if looking down on a cross section of the body at the level of the heart (Figure 2-12).

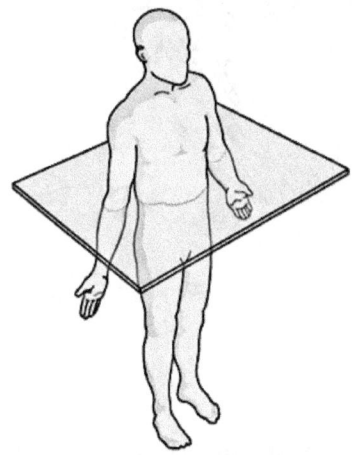

Figure 2-12. Horizontal plane.

Left ventricular muscle mass is much greater than right ventricular muscle mass and as a result the forces of left ventricular depolarization normally mask those of right ventricular depolarization.

Generation of the depolarization wave of the ventricles is shown schematically in Figure 2-13. Leads V_1 and V_2 monitor the electrical activity of the heart from the right side, V_3 and V_4 from the anterior aspect, and V_5 and V_6 from the left side. It should be noted that leads V_1 and V_6 essentially monitor the electrical activity from opposite sides of the heart, hence registering reciprocal voltages. The QRS complexes in these two leads develop during depolarization as follows: Since initial myocardial depolarization occurs in the septum from left to right (small arrow), the electrical signal travels toward V_1 and away from V_6, causing an initial small upward deflection in V_1 and a downward deflection in V_6. After septal depolarization, the wave sweeps downward around the lower part of the heart and then back up the myocardium (large arrow) away from V_1 and toward V_6, causing a downward deflection in V_1 and an upward deflection in V_6. As depolarization is completed, the recording returns to baseline.

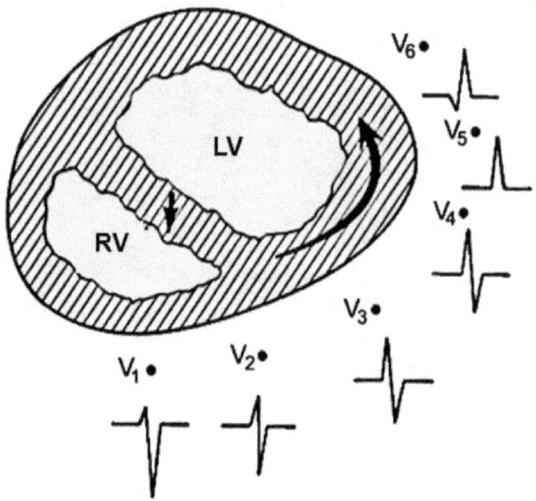

Figure 2-13. QRS waves in the six chest leads. The recorded signal becomes positive as the depolarization wave moves toward an electrode and negative as it moves away from an electrode.

R Wave Progression

Lead V_1 normally consists of a small R wave and a large S wave, whereas lead V_6 consists of a small Q wave and a large R wave (Figure 2-14). Since V_3 and V_4 are located midway between V_1 and V_6, the QRS complex would be expected to be nearly isoelectric in one of these leads; that is, the positive deflection and the negative deflection will be about equal. The magnitude of the deflection of V_2 is between that of V_1 and V_3 and the magnitude of the deflection of V_5 is between that of V_4 and V_6. Hence, a progression of the R wave occurs, getting progressively more positive from V_1 to V_6. R wave progression may be abnormal in anterior myocardial infarction.

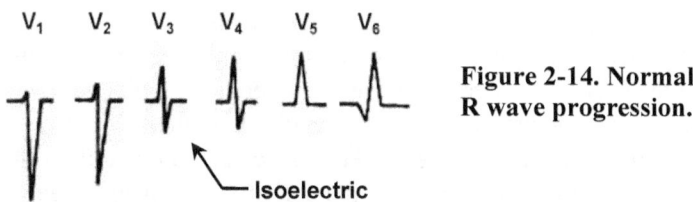

Figure 2-14. Normal
R wave progression.

Other causes of poor R wave progression include:

- Congenital heart disease
- Dextrocardia
- Lead misplacement
- Left bundle branch block or left anterior fascicular block
- Left ventricular hypertrophy
- Old anterior myocardial infarction
- Tension pneumothorax (mediastinal shift)
- Wolff-Parkinson-White syndrome

Lead Combinations

The various limb and chest leads can be grouped in combinations depending on the anatomical area of the heart they monitor.

- **Lateral leads.** The lateral leads (I, aV_L, V_5-V_6) monitor the electrical activity of the lateral aspect of the heart.
- **Inferior (diaphragmatic) leads.** The inferior leads (II, III, aV_F) monitor the electrical activity of the underside of the heart.
- **Anterior leads.** The anterior leads (V_3 and V_4) monitor the electrical activity of the anterior aspect of the heart.
- **Right leads.** The right leads (V_1 and V_2) monitor the electrical activity of the right side of the heart and the septum

NORMAL ELECTROCARDIOGRAM

Mean Electrical Activity

The *QRS axis* is the "average" direction of electrical activity during ventricular depolarization (*mean electrical activity*). The mean electrical axis may shift due to physical change in the position of the heart, chamber hypertrophy, or conduction block.

The mean electrical activity of ventricular depolarization in the frontal plane can be represented by a vector. The length of this vector indicates the magnitude of the activity. The mean direction of the depolarization wave is represented by the angle of the vector in regard to the six limb leads.

In Figure 2-15, the mean vector is determined from the magnitudes of the QRS voltages in leads I and aV_F. The normal mean vector is between -30 and 90 degrees, averaging 58 degrees as shown. The mean vector can be determined using the magnitudes of QRS complexes in other leads to project lines at 90 degrees from their tips to a crossing point, which is the tip of the mean vector.

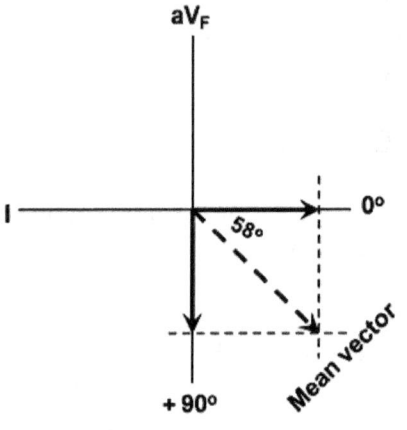

Figure 2-15. The normal mean vector of ventricular depolarization as determined from the QRS magnitudes in leads I and aV_F.

Parameters of the Normal ECG

A normal 12-lead electrocardiogram is shown in Figure 2-16. A *rhythm strip* is displayed along the bottom. Parameters associated with a normal electrocardiogram include:

- Pulse rate is between 60 and 100 beats per minute (bpm).
- Rhythm is regular except for minor variations with breathing (usually no more than 10 percent increase during inhalation).
- A P wave precedes every QRS complex. P waves should be

upright in leads I, II and V_3-V_6. It is normally negative in lead aV_R and may be biphasic in leads V_1 and V_2. If the P wave is not upright in leads I and II and negative in lead aV_R suspect that normal sinus rhythm is not present.

- PR interval is the time required for completion of atrial depolarization; conduction through the AV note, bundle of His, and bundle branches; and arrival at the ventricular myocardial cells. The normal PR interval is 0.12 to 0.20 seconds.

- The QRS interval represents the time required for ventricular cells to depolarize. The normal duration is 0.06 to 0.10 seconds.

- The QT interval is inversely proportional to the heart rate. At normal heart rates it lasts between 0. 34 and 0.42 seconds. QTc can be determined by Hodge's formula or other formulas. QTc should not be more than 0.44 seconds in males and 0.46 seconds in females.

- aV_R, for practical purposes, is an upside-down version of lead I.

- The QRS deflections in leads I and III approximately equal that of lead II. Similarly, the sum of The QRS deflections in leads aV_R, aV_L, and aV_F should approximately equal zero. When this is not true, there is reason to suspect the electrodes were placed incorrectly or that recordings were mixed up during mounting.

- Good R wave progression occurs in the chest leads, with the transition zone (point of equal positive and negative voltages) occurring somewhere between V_3 and V_4.

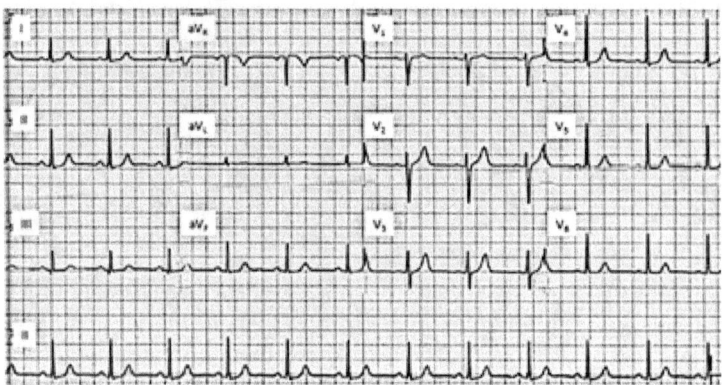

Figure 2-16. A normal ECG.

Chapter 2 Quiz

1. Determine QT
2. Calculate QTc.
3. Is the QTc normal or prolonged?

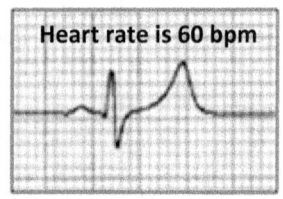

4. Is the R wave progression normal or abnormal?

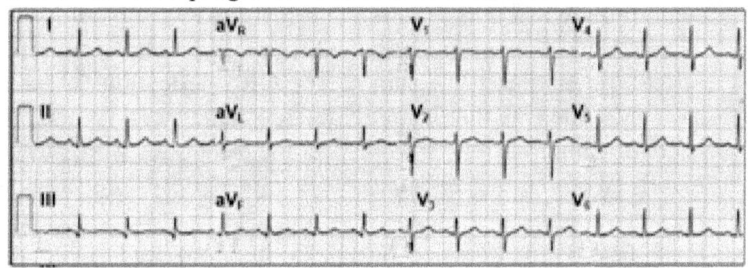

5. Locate the placements of the
chest leads.

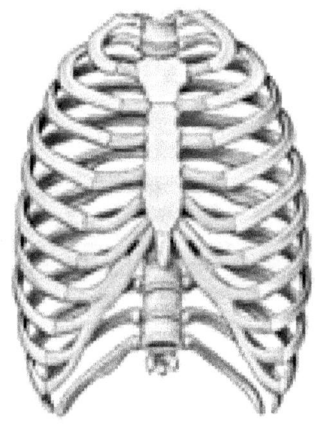

Are the following unipolar or bipolar leads?
   6. Standard limb leads
   7. Augmented limb leads
   8. Precordial leads

Name the
leads (ques-
tions 9,10,11)

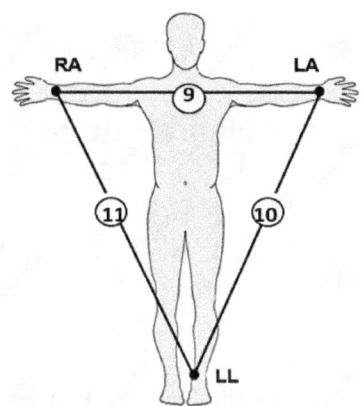

12. What four leads make up the lateral leads?

13. What three leads make up the Inferior (diaphragmatic) leads?

14. What two chest leads make up the strictly anterior leads?

15. What two chest leads make up the right leads?

16. The normal mean vector axis is approximately:
   A. 90°
   B. 120°
   C. 30°
   D. 60°

Chapter 3

Heart Rate and Axis

HEART RATE

A normal *heart rate* is defined as 60 to 100 bpm. The rate is normally set by the rhythm of the sinoatrial (SA) node, which is located in the posterior wall of the right atrium. When the sinoatrial node fails to function as the pacemaker, another area of the heart assumes the pacemaker role. This site may be another area of the atria, the atrioventricular (AV) node, or an area of the ventricles. When an area of the atria other than the sinoatrial node becomes the pacemaker, the rate is usually about the same as that of the sinoatrial node. Should the atrioventricular node become the pacemaker, the rate will be about 60 bpm. If an area of the ventricles assumes the role, the heart rate will be 30 to 40 beats/minute.

Heart rate can be estimated in a straight-forward fashion from an electrocardiogram tracing (Figure 3-1). The RR interval is inversely proportional to heart rate. At a normal paper speed of 25 mm per second, an RR interval of 0.2 seconds (one large square) indicates a rate of 300 bpm. An RR interval of two large squares indicates a rate half as fast, or 150 bpm. Similarly, three large squares indicate 100 bpm, four large squares indicate 75 bpm, five large squares indicate 60 bpm, and six large squares indicate 50 bpm. In other words, heart rate can be determined by dividing 300 by the number of large squares.

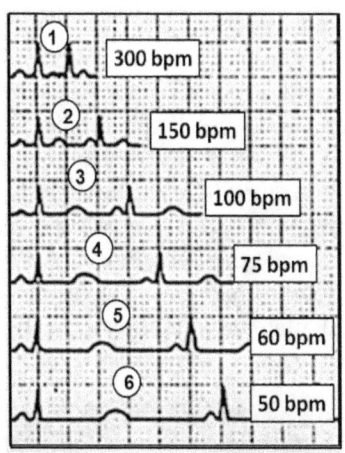

Figure 3-1. Heart rates between 50 and 300 bpm can be estimated from the number of large squares in an RR interval.

Heart rates of less than 50 bpm are estimated as follows: The electrocardiogram has small vertical markings above the graph portion at three-second intervals. Heart rate is estimated by multiplying the number and portions of cycles in a six-second interval by ten. For example, if there are 3-1/2 cycles in a six-second interval, the heart rate is 35 bpm (3-1/2 x 10 = 35). Some examples of heart rates of less than 50 bpm are shown in Figure 3-2.

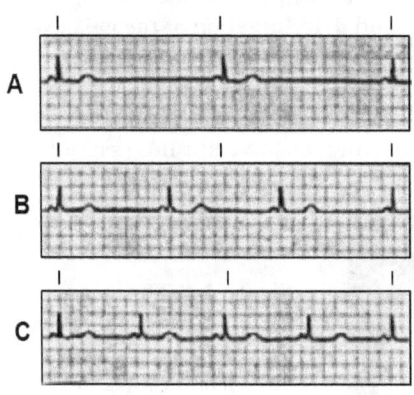

Figure 3-2. Heart rates less than 50 bpm can be estimated with the aid of markings at three-second intervals along the top of the graph paper: (A) 20 bpm, (B) 30 bpm, and (C) 40 bpm.

AXIS

Axis refers to the direction of the mean vector of ventricular depolarization. Two methods for determining the axis of the mean vector are (1) the vector method and (2) the isoelectric method.

Vector Method

As an example of the vector method let us consider the following vectors in leads I and aV$_F$ (Figure 3-3). For lead I the net QRS is +7 little squares and for lead aV$_F$ it is 6 little squares. Lines (dashed) are drawn at 90° to these vectors. The point where the two dashed lines cross is the tip of the mean vector. Knowing two sides (6,7) of a right triangle we can calculate the hypotenuse (mean vector magnitude) using the Pythagorean theorem. The result is 9.2. Also, by trigonometry, we can calculate the direction to be 49.3 degrees from the horizontal.

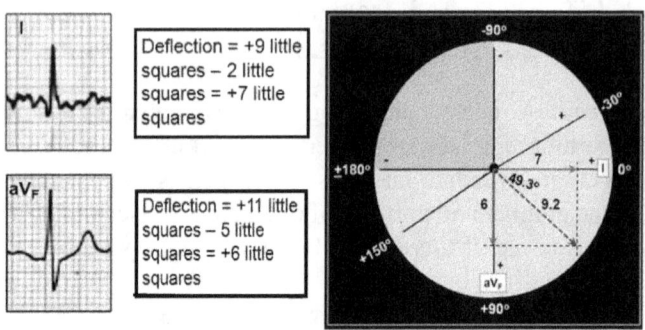

Figure 3-3. Calculations of the sum of the positive and the negative deflections of the QRS complex and determination of the mean vector.

It's extremely rare that we need to be this exact. We need only determine in which range or zone the mean vector lies (Figure 3-4).

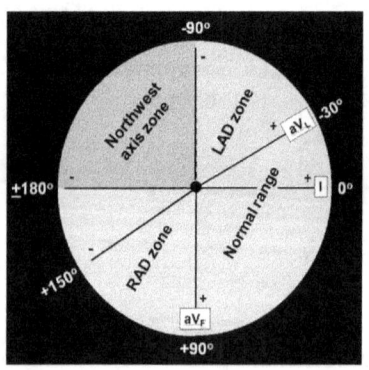

Figure 3-4. The mean vector of ventricular depolarization may fall in the normal range, the LAD zone, the RAD zone, or the Northwest axis zone.

To determine the range or zone we go through a series of steps known as three-lead analysis (leads I, II, and aV$_F$).

1. Check to see if the mean vector is in the **normal range** (+90° to -30°). If not,
2. Check to see if the mean vector is in the **left axis deviation zone** (-30° to -90°). If not,
3. Check to see if it is in the **right axis deviation zone** (+90° to +180°). If not,
4. Check to see if it is in the **Northwest axis zone** (- 90° to- 180°).

Actually, these can be done in any order.

Determining the axis of the mean vector involves the inspection of leads I, II, and aV$_F$.

Normal Range

If the mean vector is in the normal range (+90° to -30°), both leads I and II will be positive; that is, the sum of the positive and the negative deflections of the QRS complexes will be positive (Figure 3-5).

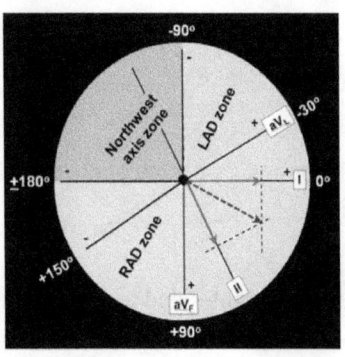

Figure 3-5. Normal range: Both leads I and II are positive

If the mean vector is in the normal range, we are finished with mean vector determination. Record it as normal.

Left Axis Deviation Zone

If the axis of the mean vector is not in the normal range, check to see if it is in the left axis deviation zone (-30° to -90°). Lead I will be positive and lead II will be negative (Figure 3-6).

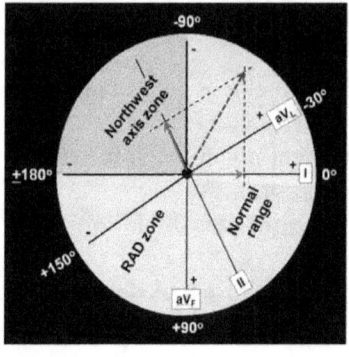

Figure 3-6. Left axis deviation: Lead I is positive and lead II is negative.

Causes of left axis deviation include:

- Emphysema
- Hyperkalemia
- Hypertension
- Left anterior hemiblock
- Left bundle branch block
- Left ventricular hypertrophy
- Ostium primum atrial septal defect
- Past anterior myocardial infarction
- Subaortic stenosis
- Valvular heart disease (aortic stenosis or regurgitation, mitral regurgitation, tricuspid atresia)
- Ventricular pacing
- Wolff-Parkinson-White syndrome (right-sided accessory pathway)

Right Axis Deviation Zone

If the mean vector is not in the left axis deviation zone, check to see if it is in the right axis deviation zone. This means that the mean vector will be between +90 degrees and +180 degrees: Thus, lead I will be negative and lead aV$_F$ will be positive (Figure 3-7).

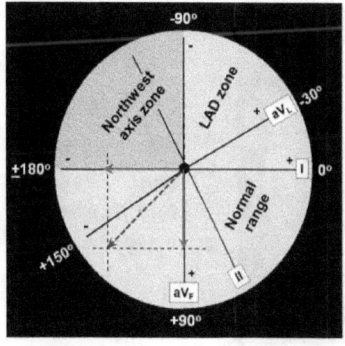

Figure 3-7. Right axis deviation. If lead I is negative and lead aV$_F$ is positive, the mean vector is in the RAD zone.

Causes of right axis deviation include:

- Acute pulmonary embolus (sudden shift to the right)
- Anterolateral myocardial infarction
- Atrial septal defect
- Chronic lung disease (emphysema, chronic bronchitis)
- Dextrocardia
- Left posterior hemiblock
- Normal finding in children and tall thin adults
- Reversed arm leads
- Right ventricular hypertrophy
- Ventricular septal defect
- Wolff-Parkinson-White syndrome with left-sided accessory pathway

Northwest Axis Zone

If the mean vector is not in the right axis deviation zone, check to see if it is in the Northwest axis zone (-90° to -180°) as shown in Figure 3-8. Both leads I and aV$_F$ will be negative. Other names for Northwest axis zone are "no man's land" and "extreme Axis."

The problem with this zone is that it may represent either an extreme RAD or an extreme LAD. The important thing is to recognize that it is abnormal and most often is either a left hemiblock or right ventricular hypertrophy. An axis in this zone is unusual.

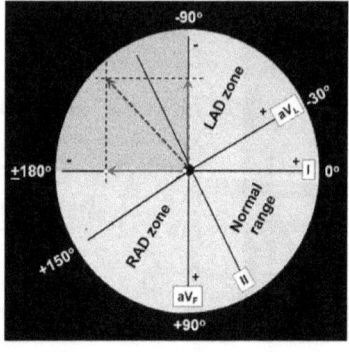

Figure 3-8. Northwest axis zone: Leads I and aV$_F$ are negative.

Other causes of Northwest axis are:

- Artificial cardiac pacing
- Severe emphysema
- Hyperkalemia
- Accidental lead transposition
- Ventricular tachycardia

Normal Zone and Gray Zone

It sometimes is desirable to subdivide the normal range into the normal zone and the gray zone because it gives us information that the mean vector, if in the gray zone, is approaching left axis deviation (Figure 3-9).

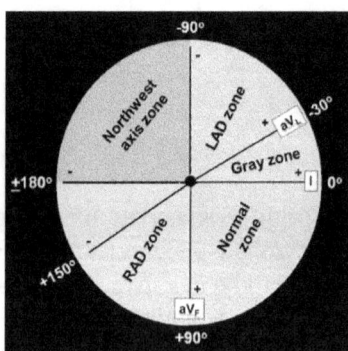

Figure 3-9. Subdivision of the Normal Range into the Normal Zone and the Gray Zone.

Normal Zone. The normal zone lies between 0° and +90°. Both leads I and aV$_F$ are positive as illustrated in Figure 3-10.

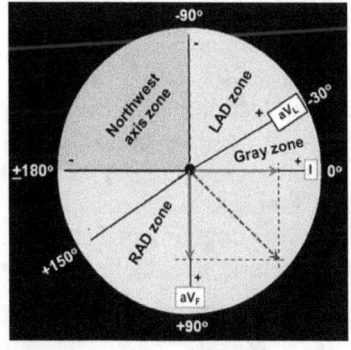

Figure 3-10. Normal Zone. Leads I and aV$_F$ are positive.

Gray Zone. The gray zone lies between 0° and -30° (Figure 3-11). If the mean vector is in the normal range, but not in the normal zone then it must be in the gray zone. That is, if leads I and II are positive and lead aV$_F$ is negative, then the mean vector is in the gray zone.

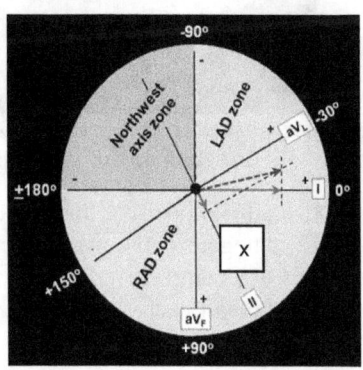

Figure 3-11. Gray zone: Both leads I and II are positive and lead aV$_F$ is negative.

The criteria for axis determination are given in Table 3-1.

Table 3-1. Summary of the vector method for axis determination

	Lead I	Lead II	Lead aV$_F$
Normal Range	+	+	
LAD Zone	+	-	
RAD Zone	-		+
Norwest Axis Zone	-		-
Normal Zone	+		+
Gray Zone	+	+	-

Isoelectric Method

A second method for determining axis is the *isoelectric method*. In this method we look for a limb lead in which the QRS complex is isoelectric (negative deflection = positive deflection). The axis of the mean vector must be at an angle of 90 degrees to this lead. For example, if the QRS complex in lead II is isoelectric (Figure 3-13A), the mean vector must be in the direction of lead aV_L, either -30° or +150° (Figure 3-13B). To determine which, we must look

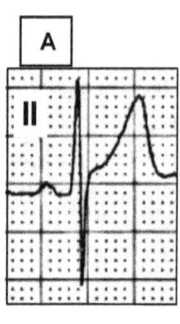 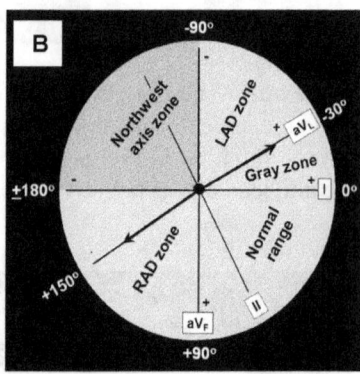

Figure 3-13. (A) The QRS complex is isoelectric in lead II. (B) The mean vector either points in the -30° direction or the +150° direction

at another lead. For instance, If lead I is positive, the mean vector must point toward -30°. If lead I is negative, the mean vector must point toward +150°. Suppose the QRS complex in lead I is negative (Figure 3-14A), then the axis of the mean vector points in the +150° direction (Figure 3-14B).

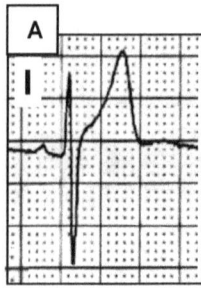 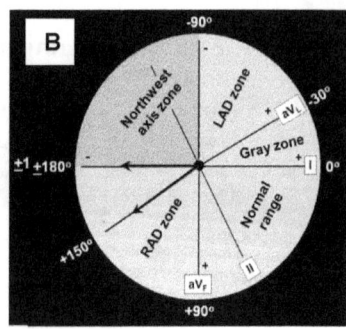

Figure 3-14. When the QRS complex in lead II is isoelectric and the QRS complex in lead I is negative (A), the mean vector of ventricular depolarization points in the +150° direction (B).

The problem inherent in this method is that an isoelectric lead may not be present.

Chapter 3 Quiz

1. What is the heart rate?

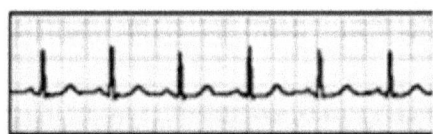

2. What is the heart rate?

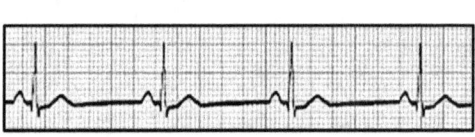

3. What is the heart rate?

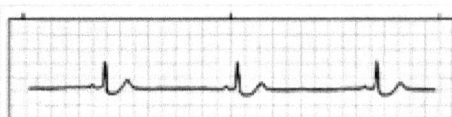

4. Determine QT

5. Calculate QTc using Hodge's formula

$$QTc = QT + 0.00175(\text{heart rate} - 60)$$

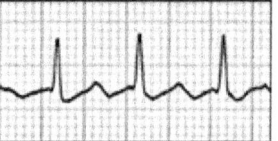

6. In which zone is the mean vector (normal range, LAD zone, RAD zone, NW axis zone, normal zone, gray zone)?

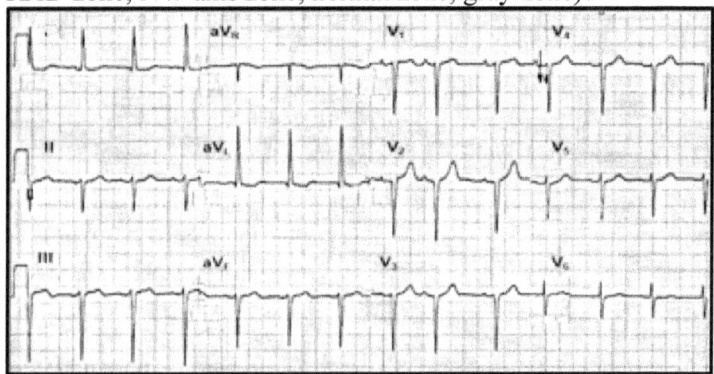

7. In which zone is the mean vector (normal range, LAD zone, RAD zone, NW axis zone, normal zone, gray zone)?

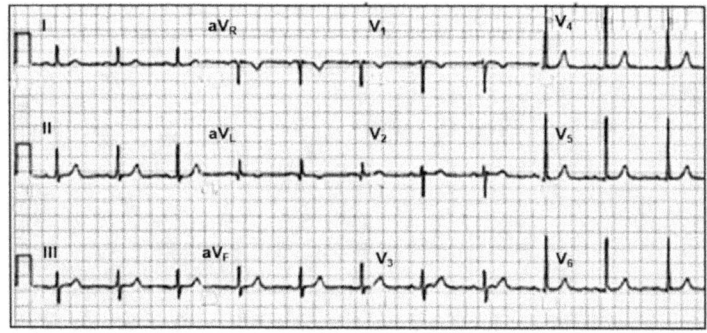

8. In which zone is the mean vector (normal range, LAD zone, RAD zone, NW axis zone, normal zone, gray zone)?

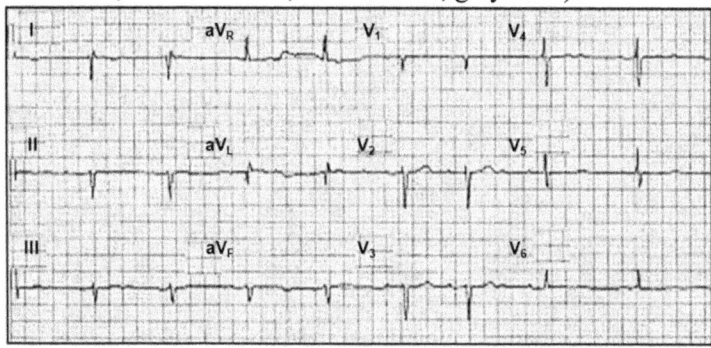

9. In which zone is the mean vector (normal range, LAD zone, RAD zone, NW axis zone, normal zone, gray zone)?

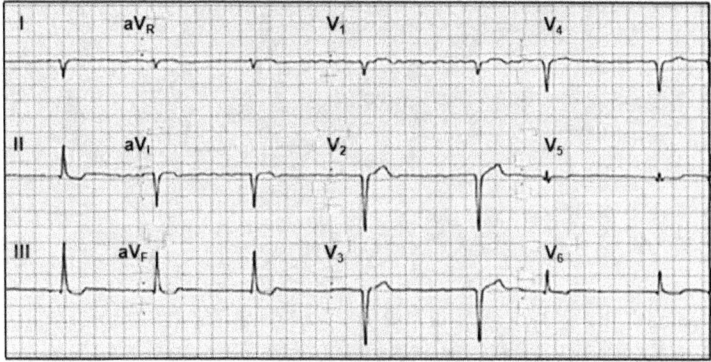

10. In which zone is the mean vector (normal range, LAD zone, RAD zone, NW axis zone, normal zone, gray zone)?

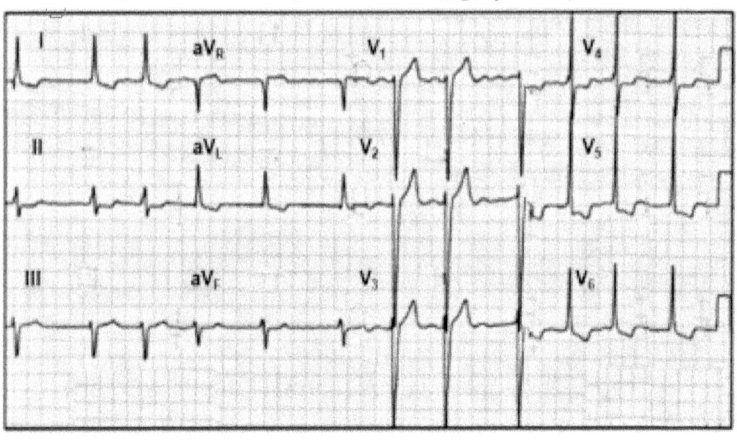

Chapter 4

Atrial Enlargement, Ventricular Hypertrophy, and Hypertrophic Cardiomyopathy

ATRIAL ENLARGEMENT

Atrial depolarization is reflected in the P wave of the electrocardiogram. The normal P wave is less than 2.5 mm high and is 0.08 to 0.11 seconds in duration. Because lead V_1 is the closest to the atria, it gives the most accurate information about atrial enlargement. Lead II is very a useful lead to observe because it is approximately parallel to the forces of atrial depolarization.

The right atrium is responsible for the left-hand portion of the P wave and the left atrium for the right-hand portion (Figure 4-1).

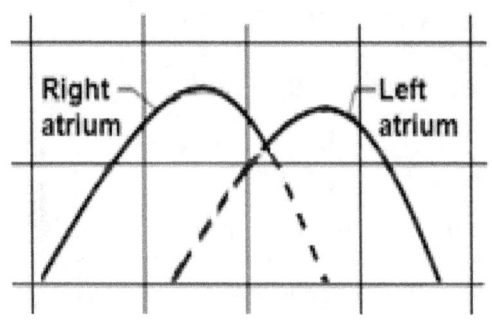

Figure 4-1. Contributions of the right and left atria to the P wave.

Right Atrial Enlargement

Criteria for *right atrial enlargement (RAE)* include:

- P wave is greater than 2.5 mm tall in leads II, III, or aV$_F$ or P wave is greater than 1.5 mm in lead V$_1$
- The positive part of the biphasic P wave in lead V$_1$ is larger than the negative part.
- The width of the P wave is usually normal

P wave configurations from leads II and V$_1$ provide clues to right atrial enlargement (Figure 4-2).

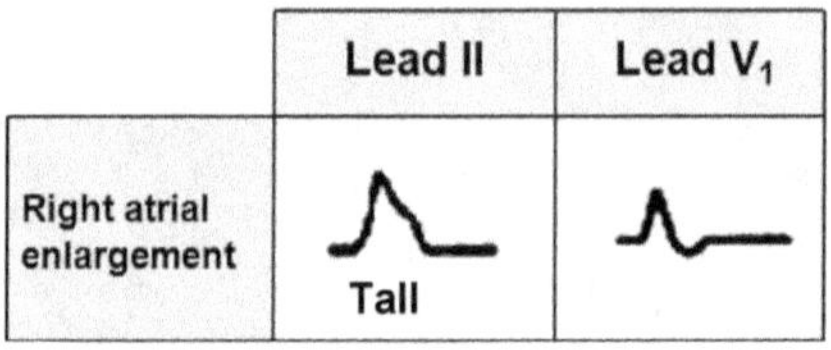

	Lead II	Lead V₁
Right atrial enlargement	∧ Tall	∧

Figure 4-2. P wave configurations from leads II and V₁ provide clues to right atrial enlargement.

The accuracy of RAE criteria is greatly improved in the presence of right ventricular hypertrophy.

Right atrial enlargement may occur in a variety of clinical settings, including:

- Right ventricular hypertrophy
- Pulmonary disease (emphysema, chronic bronchitis)
- Heart disease (pulmonary stenosis, atrial septal defect, mitral stenosis or regurgitation, tetralogy of Fallot).

Because RAE is so frequently seen in chronic pulmonary disease, the peaked P wave is often called *P pulmonale.*

Left Atrial Enlargement

Criteria for *left atrial enlargement (LAE)* include:

- The P wave length in lead II is greater than 0.12 seconds in duration or the terminal downward deflection of the P wave in lead V₁ is greater than 0.04 seconds in length and greater than 1

millimeter negative deflection
- Bifid P wave in lead II with the second portion greater than the first
- Enlarged terminal negative portion of the P wave in V_1.

P wave configurations from leads II and V_1 provide clues to left atrial enlargement (Figure 4-3).

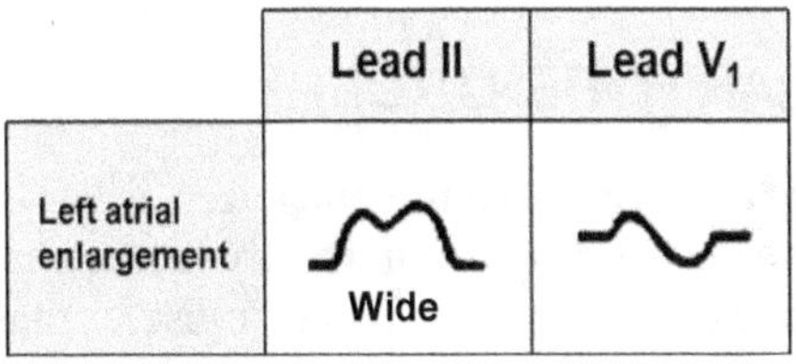

	Lead II	Lead V₁
Left atrial enlargement	Wide	

Figure 4-3. P wave configurations from leads II and V_1 provide clues to left atrial enlargement

Left atrial enlargement occurs in a variety of clinical settings. It may be secondary to:

- Left ventricular enlargement (congestive heart failure, hypertensive heart disease, aortic stenosis or regurgitation)
- Mitral valve disease (stenosis, regurgitation).

Because LAE is so frequently seen with mitral valve disease, a broad notched P wave is often called *P mitrale*.

Left atrial enlargement is a significant risk factor for developing atrial fibrillation.

Biatrial Enlargement

Biatrial enlargement (BAE) has features of both RAE and LAE. Biatrial enlargement presents with

- A P wave amplitude > 2.5 mm and a duration of > 0.12 seconds in lead II.
- A large biphasic P wave in lead V_1 with the initial component greater than 1.5 mm in height and the terminal component at least 1 mm in depth and 0.04 seconds in duration.

P wave configurations from leads II and V_1 provide clues to biatrial enlargement (Figure 4-4).

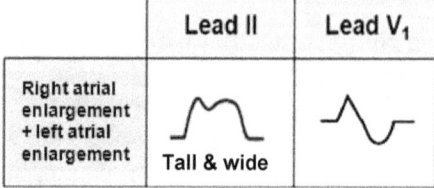

	Lead II	Lead V₁
Right atrial enlargement + left atrial enlargement	Tall & wide	

Figure 4-4. P wave configurations from leads II and V₁ provide clues to biatrial enlargement.

VENTRICULAR HYPERTROPHY

Ventricular hypertrophy can occur in the right ventricle, left ventricle, or both ventricles. The electrocardiogram normally reflects left ventricular depolarization because left ventricular muscle mass is much greater than right ventricular muscle mass. However, when right ventricular muscle mass becomes great enough, it causes alterations in the positivity of the right chest leads of the electrocardiogram that can be interpreted as right ventricular hypertrophy.

Right Ventricular Hypertrophy

In the absence of myocardial infarction or right bundle branch block, the diagnosis of *right ventricular hypertrophy* (RVH) can be made when:

- R > than S in lead V_1 o r V_2 or S > than R in lead V_5 or V_6
- R wave in lead V_1 + S wave in lead V_5 or $V_6 \geq 11$ mm

An example of RVH is given in Figure 4-5.

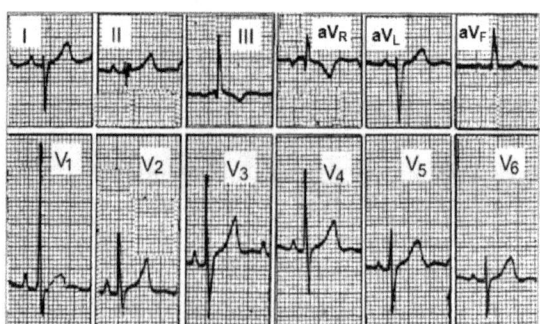

Figure 4-5. Right ventricular hypertrophy. Note the presence of RAD and R > S in V_1 and the R wave in V_1 + the S wave in $V_5 \geq 11$ mm.

Right ventricular hypertrophy occurs in a variety of clinical conditions, including:

- Chronic pulmonary diseases (emphysema, chronic bronchitis, cystic fibrosis)
- Congenital heart disease (pulmonary stenosis, atrial septal defect, tetralogy of Fallot)
- High altitude
- Pulmonary hypertension secondary to mitral stenosis
- Ventricular septal defect

Other causes of an R/S ratio >1 in lead V_1 include:

- Posterior wall myocardial infarction, which also causes ST segment depression in V_1-V_3, but T waves are symmetrically inverted and the patient presents with symptoms
- Right bundle branch block
- Wolff-Parkinson-White syndrome
- Lead misplacement (V_1 is placed too high)
- Isolated posterior wall hypertrophy (occurs in Duchenne's muscular dystrophy)

Left Ventricular Hypertrophy

Left ventricular hypertrophy (LVH) causes an increase in the height and depth of the QRS complexes. Several criteria, based on chest leads or limb leads, have been developed. These criteria are more accurate for individuals greater than or equal to 35 years of age. Two of these criteria are as follow:

- ***Sokolow-Lyon Criteria***: If the sum of the S wave in V_1 and the R wave in V_5 or V_6 is > 35 mm or the R wave in aV_L is ≥ 11 mm, then LVH may be present.
- ***Cornell criteria***: If the sum of the R wave in aV_L and the S wave in V_3 is > 28 mm in males or > 20 mm in females, then LVH may present.

The ECG of a patient with left ventricular hypertrophy is shown in Figure 4-6.

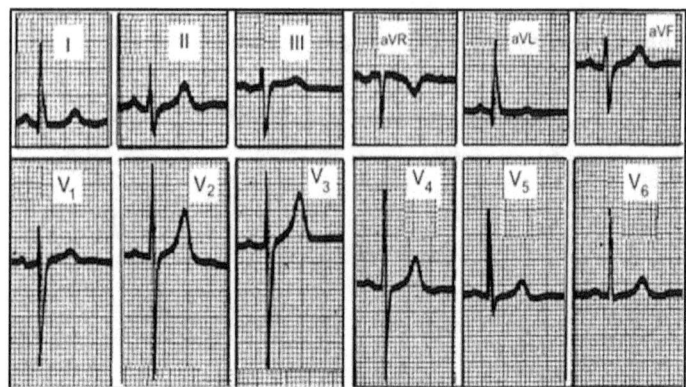

Figure 4-6. Left ventricular hypertrophy in a male. Note that the sum of the S wave in V_1 plus the R wave in V_5 or V_6 is > 35 mm and the R wave in aV_L is > 11 mm (*Sokolow-Lyon Criteria*). Also, the sum of the R wave in aV_L and the S wave in V_3 is > 28 mm (*Cornell criteria*).

The fact that one set of criteria has not universally been agreed upon means that the use of any lacks satisfactory accuracy. The diagnosis of LVH is best made by echocardiography.

Left axis deviation is often present with left ventricular hypertrophy, but is of little significance and is not considered part of the criteria for diagnosis. Signs of LAE may be present.

The electrocardiograms of thin young men often meet the criteria for left ventricular hypertrophy without ventricular hypertrophy actually being present. Individuals with emphysema or pericardial effusion may have reduced QRS voltages and, hence, masked left ventricular hypertrophy.

Ventricular hypertrophy occurs naturally as a reaction to aerobic exercise and strength training. Pathologic causes include:

- Chronic cocaine or methamphetamine use
- Hypertension
- Hypertrophic cardiomyopathy
- Valvular heart disease (aortic stenosis, aortic regurgitation, mitral regurgitation)
- Congenital heart disease

The diagnosis of LVH is made more accurately in the presence of *left ventricular systolic overload* (strain), which can be systolic or diastolic overload.

Biventricular Hypertrophy

Biventricular Hypertrophy (BVH) is a difficult ECG diagnosis to make. In the presence of LAE any one of the following suggests this diagnosis:

- Signs of both LVH and RVH on the same ECG — that is. positive diagnostic criteria for LVH with some additional features suggestive of RVH.
- Large biphasic QRS complexes in leads V₂-V₅. This is the classic ECG pattern of BVH typically seen in children with ventriculoseptal defect
- RAD may be present

Figure 4-7 shows the large biphasic QRS complexes seen in leads V₂-V₅ in children with ventriculoseptal defect.

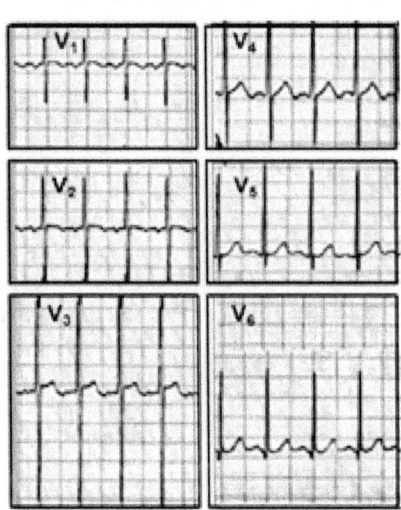

Figure 4-7. ECG from a child with a ventriculoseptal defect and biventricular hypertrophy. Note the large biphasic QRS complexes in leads V₂-V₅

Other causes of biventricular hypertrophy include:

- Metabolic storage disorders (amyloidosis, glycogen storage muscle disease)
- Congenital heart disease (patent ductus arteriosus, tetralogy of Fallot)

Ventricular Overload (Strain)

Systolic ventricular overload means that the load is so great that ventricular function is impaired. The overload can be systolic or diastolic in nature. We will limit our discussion to systolic overload.

The overload may be due to volume or pressure factors. With *volume overload* the ventricle has too large a volume of blood for it to function efficiently. With *pressure overload* the ventricle has to contract against too great a pressure for it to function efficiently.

Right Ventricular Overload (Strain)

With severe RVH overload the ECG may show signs of strain; that is, the T waves may be directed away from the QRS complexes. The chest leads of an electrocardiogram with *right ventricular systolic overload* are shown in Figure 4-8. In addition to the right ventricular hypertrophy criteria, T wave inversion and/or ST segment depression are present in the right chest leads.

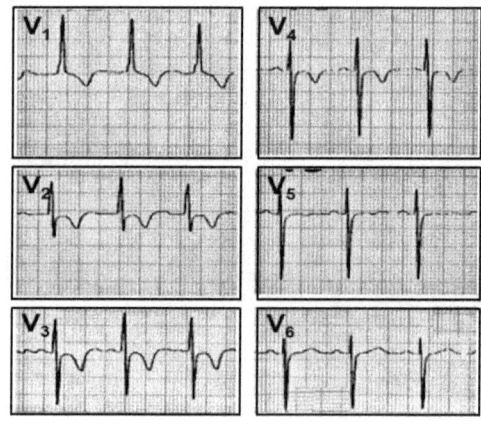

Figure 4-8. Right ventricular hypertrophy with strain. Note the R > S in V$_1$, the depressed ST segments, and the inverted T waves in the Right chest leads.

Right ventricular volume overload can be due to:

- Valvular heart disease
  - Tricuspid regurgitation
  - Pulmonary regurgitation
- Congenital heart defects
  - Atrial septal defect

Right ventricular pressure overload can be due to:

- Valvular heart disease
  - Pulmonary stenosis
- Pulmonary hypertension

Left Ventricular Overload (Strain)

In addition to the criteria for left ventricular hypertrophy, with over-load T wave inversion and/or ST segment depression occurs in the left chest leads (Figure 4-9). Left ventricular overload can be due to volume overload or pressure overload.

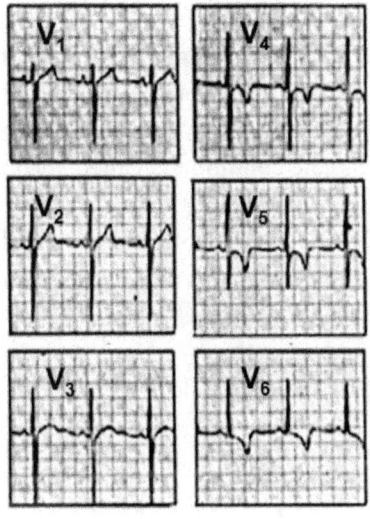

Figure 4-9. Left ventricular hypertrophy with strain. Note the large QRS complexes and the inverted T waves in the lateral chest leads.

Left ventricular volume overload can be due to:

- Valvular heart disease

- Aortic regurgitation
- Mitral regurgitation
- Congenital heart defects
  - Patent ductus arteriosus
  - Ventricular septal defect
  - Large arteriovenous malformation

Left ventricular pressure overload can be due to:

- Valvular heart disease
  - Aortic stenosis
  - Coarctation of the aorta
- Hypertension

HYPERTROPHIC CARDIOMYOPATHY

Hypertrophic cardiomyopathy (HCM) is a genetic disorder that can affect people of any age. It is a common cause of cardiac arrest in young people, especially young athletes (such as Reggie Lewis, a Boston Celtic, died of HCM at age 27).

HCM occurs when heart muscle cells enlarge and cause the walls of the left ventricle to thicken. The septum thickens and bulges into the left ventricle. The thickening may block blood flow out of the ventricle. If this happens, the condition is called *chronic hypertrophic obstructive cardiomyopathy (HOCM)*.

HCM also can affect the mitral valve, causing mitral insufficiency. The changes increase the amount of work the ventricle must do to pump blood. Symptoms can include chest pain, dizziness, shortness of breath, fainting, or sudden death.

Some ECG abnormalities due to HCM include:

- Left ventricular hypertrophy results in increased precordial voltages (left ventricular hypertrophy) and non-specific ST segment and T wave abnormalities.
- Asymmetrical septal hypertrophy produces deep, narrow, dagger-like Q waves in the lateral leads (I, aV_L, V_5-V_6,)

- Left atrial enlargement due to impaired ventricular filling may occur.

An ECG of a patient with hypertrophic cardiomyopathy is shown in Figure 4-10.

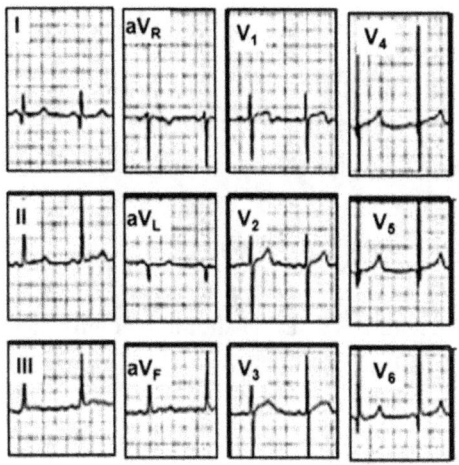

Figure 4-10. Hypertrophic cardiomyopathy. Note the large QRS complexes and the dagger-like Q waves in leads I, aV$_L$, and V$_5$-V$_6$.

The apical variant of HOM does not result in septal Q waves, as the septum is normal in thickness. The cardiac apex, however is abnormally thickened, resulting in large, diffuse T wave changes throughout the precordial leads.

CONGENITAL CORONARY ARTERY ANOMALIES

Congenital coronary artery anomalies are another cause of sudden death, particularly in young athletes (such as Pete Maravich who died after a pickup basketball game at age 40. Maravich is the all-time leading college scorer in both total points and points per game. He had a missing left coronary artery). These anomalies are observed both in pediatric and adult patients, with an equal incidence of sudden death.

Coronary artery anomalies consist of a wide range of defects, including anomalous origin, anomalous course, or both. The ECG may be normal or abnormal and depends on the specific anomaly.

Chapter 4 Quiz

1. The normal P wave is < _____ mm high.
2. The normal P wave is < _____ seconds in duration.
3. Right axis deviation is part of the criteria for right ventricular hypertrophy (T or F).
4. Left axis deviation is part of the criteria for left ventricular hypertrophy (T or F).
5. The electrocardiograpy diagnosis of LVH should be confirmed by echocardiography (T or F).

6. Right, left, or biatrial enlargement

Lead I	Lead V₁
Tall and wide	

7. Right, left, or biatrial enlargement?

Lead I	Lead V₁
Tall	

8. Right, left, or biatrial enlargement?

Lead I	Lead V₁
Wide	

9. Right, left, or biventricular hypertrophy?

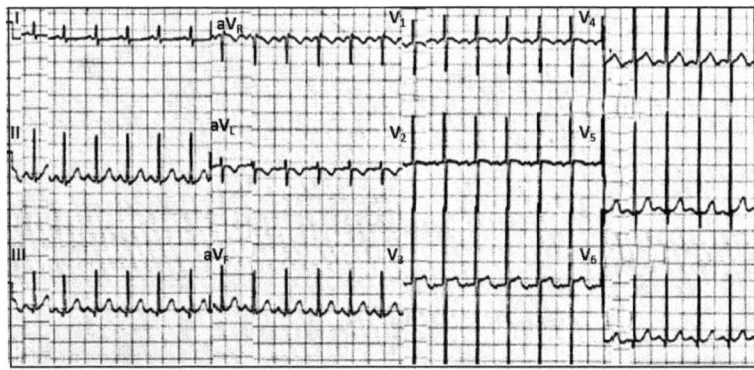

10. Right, left, or biventricular hypertrophy?

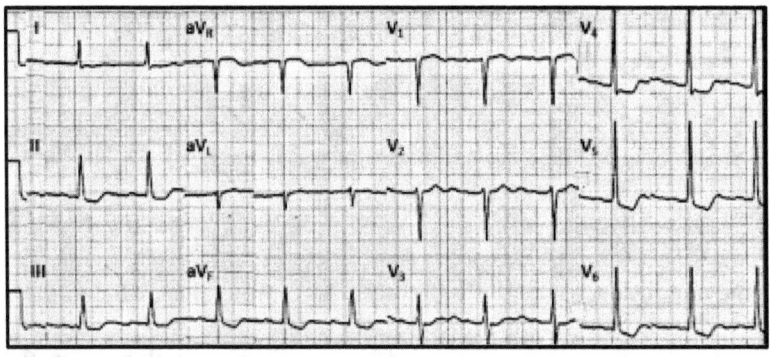

11. Right, left, or biventricular hypertrophy?

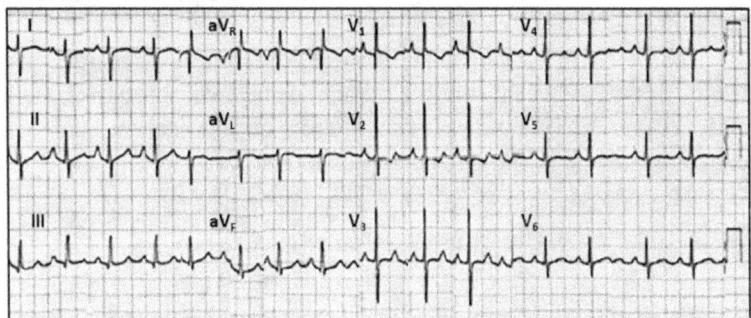

Chapter 5

Intraventricular Conduction Defects

In the normal process of depolarization, the electrical stimulus originates in the sinoatrial (SA) node, and then passes through the atria before reaching the atrioventricular (AV) node. From here it passes through the AV junction (bundle of His), which becomes the right and left bundle branches. The left bundle branch divides into the left anterior fascicle and the right posterior fascicle. The signal then spreads throughout the ventricular muscle.

Normally, the entire process of ventricular depolarization occurs in less than 0.1 seconds. Any process that interferes with normal depolarization of the ventricles may prolong the QRS complex.

Bundle branch block occurs when the signal is not conducted down the right or left bundle of the conducting pathways in the ventricles. This may occur due to degeneration with age or may be due to specific pathology, such as atherosclerosis or myocardial infarction.

Bundle branch block widens the QRS complex because electricity passes slower through cardiac muscle than through the special conducting pathways. The altered depolarization path also causes the shape of the QRS complex to change.

BUNDLE BRANCH BLOCKS

Bundle branch blocks involve either the right bundle branch or the left bundle branch after they divide from the bundle of His (AV bundle).

Right Bundle Branch Block

Blockage of conduction in the right bundle branch results in delayed depolarization of the right ventricle. The sequence of ventricular depolarization in *right bundle branch block (RBBB)* is shown in Figure 5-1. Septal depolarization is normally initiated by a branch of the left bundle branch and, hence, occurs from left to right, resulting in a small R wave in lead V_1. This is unchanged by RBBB. After septal depolarization, left ventricular depolarization takes place in a normal fashion, causing an S wave in lead V_1. Delayed depolarization of the right ventricle produces a second R wave in lead V_1 known as R′.

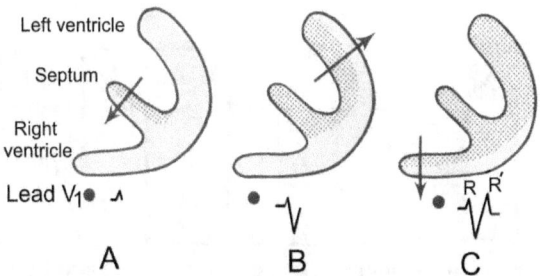

Figure 5-1. Sequence of ventricular depolarization in right bundle branch block. (A) Septal depolarization results in a small R wave in lead V_1. (B) Left ventricular depolarization results in an S wave in V_1. (C) Right ventricular depolarization produces a second R wave (R′) in lead V_1.

The ECG criteria for right bundle branch block include:

- QRS duration > 0.12 seconds.
- RR′ (RSR′) pattern in the right precordial leads V_1 or V_2 often present.
- The QRS complex in lead V_1 is upwardly deflected.
- Small S waves in leads I and aV_L

RBBB may be seen with:

- Chronically high right ventricular pressure (cor pulmonale)

- Acutely high right ventricular pressure (pulmonary embolism)

- Myocardial ischemia or infarction

- Myocardial inflammation (myocarditis)

- Hypertension

- Cardiomyopathy

- Congenital heart disease (atrial septal defect)

- Idiopathic progressive cardiac conduction disease

ECG changes of RBBB are shown in Figure 5-2.

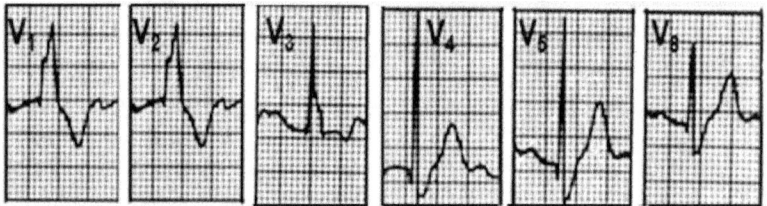

Figure 5-2. Electrocardiogram tracings typical of right bundle branch block. Note the wide QRS complexes and the RR' configuration and positively deflected QRS complexes in leads V₁ and V₂.

Left Bundle Branch Block

Blockage of conduction in the left bundle branch, prior to its bifurcation into anterior and posterior fascicles, results in delayed depolarization of the left ventricle. The sequence of ventricular depolarization with *left bundle branch block (LBBB)* is shown in Figure 5-3. The septum depolarizes from right to left since its depolarization is now initiated by the right bundle branch. Next, the right ventricle depolarizes, followed by delayed depolarization of the left ventricle, giving an RR' configuration in lead V₅ or V₆ and a QRS interval equal to or greater than 0.12 seconds.

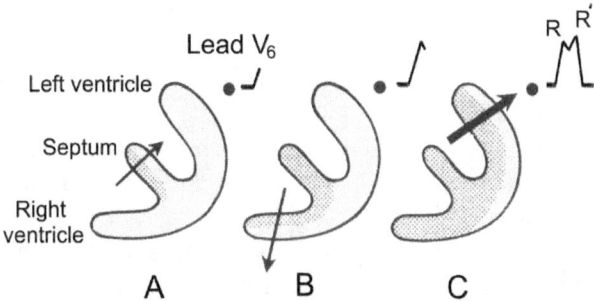

Figure 5-3. Sequence of ventricular depolarization in left bundle branch block. (A) Septal depolarization initiated by the right bundle branch occurs from right to left. (B) Right ventricular depolarization. (C) Left ventricular depolarization.

The ECG criteria for left bundle branch block (LBBB) include:

- QRS duration of $\geq$ 0.12 seconds
- Absence of Q wave in leads I, V_5, and V_6.
- ST and T wave displacements often are opposite in direction to the major deflection of the QRS complex
- RR' configuration often present in leads V_5 or V_6
- The QRS complex in lead V_1 is downwardly deflected.

An example of LBBB is shown in Figure 5-4.

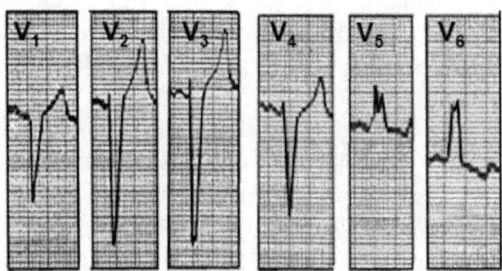

Figure 5-4. Electrocardiogram tracing typical of left bundle branch block. Note the wide QRS complexes, ST and T wave displacement in opposite direction to the QRS complexes, RR' configuration in the lateral chest leads, and negative QRS deflection in lead V_1.

Unlike RBBB, which is occasionally seen in normal subjects,

LBBB is always a sign of organic heart disease. LBBB is seen in:

- Chronic degenerative changes in the ventricular conduction system (elderly patients)
- Long-standing hypertension or valvular lesions, such as aortic stenosis or aortic regurgitation, that produce chronic strain on the left ventricle
- Coronary artery disease, since the blood supply to the conduction system arises from the coronary arteries
- Myocardial infarction

INCOMPLETE BUNDLE BRANCH BLOCK

- ***Incomplete right bundle branch block*** shows the same QRS pattern as RBBB; however, the QRS duration is between 0.1 and 0.12 seconds.
- ***Incomplete left bundle branch block*** shows the same QRS pattern as LBBB; however, the QRS duration is between 0.1 and 0.12 seconds.

HEMIBLOCKS

The two branches of the left bundle may be blocked individually. When only one branch is blocked, this is called *hemiblock—either left anterior hemiblock (LAH)* or *left posterior hemiblock (LPH)*, depending on whether the anterior or posterior fascicle is involved. The main effect of a hemiblock is to markedly change the QRS axis without changing the shape or duration of the QRS wave form.

- ***Left Anterior Hemiblock*** results in left axis deviation. In addition, there may be a small Q wave in lead I and a small R wave in lead III.
- ***Left Posterior Hemiblock*** results in right axis deviation. In addition, there may be a small R wave in lead I and a small Q wave in lead III.

LAH is relatively common, while LPH is less common. In general, findings of isolated hemiblock are of little clinical significance except when found with acute myocardial infarction. In the presence of an acute myocardial infarction, hemiblock increases the risk of death.

Hemiblock should be considered only after more common causes of axis deviation have been ruled out.

BIFASCICULAR AND TRIFASICULAR BLOCKS

Bifascicular Block

Blockage of one of the subdivisions of the left bundle branch in the presence of RBBB can occur and is known as *bifasicular block*. The configuration of the QRS complex of RBBB is not altered by left anterior or left posterior hemiblock.

RBBB plus LAH produces an electrocardiographic picture of RBBB with left axis deviation. Similarly, *RBBB plus LPH* produces an electrocardiographic picture of RBBB with right axis deviation. These combinations are potentially significant since the presence of either means the ventricles are being depolarized via only one fascicle of the left bundle branch and is subject to complete heart block.

Trifascicular Block

A trifascicular block is the combination of a right bundle branch block, left anterior or left posterior fascicular block, and a first-degree AV block. Many patients with a trifascicular block will need a permanent pacemaker because trifascicular block often becomes a third-degree block.

NONSPECIFIC INTRAVENTRICULAR CONDUCTION DEFECTS

Nonspecific intraventricular conduction defects (NIVCDs) have a QRS duration greater than 0.10 seconds, indicating slowed conduction in the ventricles. However, criteria for specific bundle branch or fascicular blocks are not met.

Chapter 5 Quiz

1. The part of the ventricle that normally depolarizes first is the right ventricle, left ventricle, or septum?

2. The septum normally depolarizes from a branch of the right bundle branch or left bundle branch?

3. The RR' pattern for RBBB occurs in the left or right chest leads?

4. The RR' pattern for LBBB occurs in the left or right chest leads?

5. If the QRS complex in lead V_1 is upwardly deflected and has a wide QRS, then a right or left bundle branch block is present?

6. If the QRS complex in lead V_1 is downwardly deflected and has a wide QRS, then a right or left bundle branch block is present?

7. Left anterior hemiblock (blockage of the left anterior fascicle) results in left or right axis deviation?

8. Left posterior hemiblock (blockage of the left posterior fascicle) results in left or right axis deviation?

9. Finding of an isolated hemiblock is indicates significant clinical pathology (T or F).

Some ECGs to interpret. Use the 8 steps discussed in Chapter 1.

10. Intraventricular Conduction Defect. Your diagnosis?

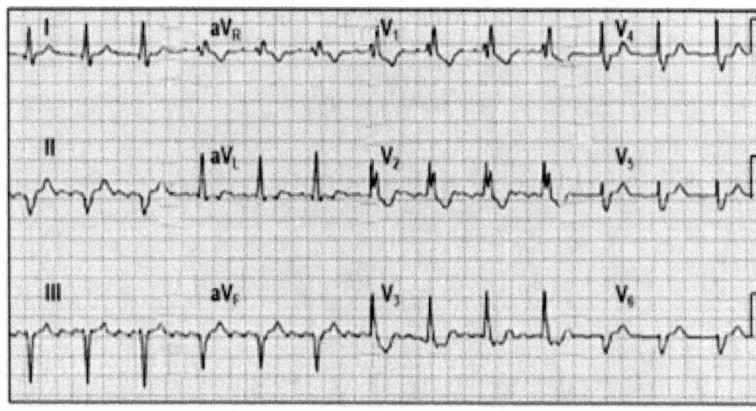

11. Intraventricular Conduction Defect. Your diagnosis?

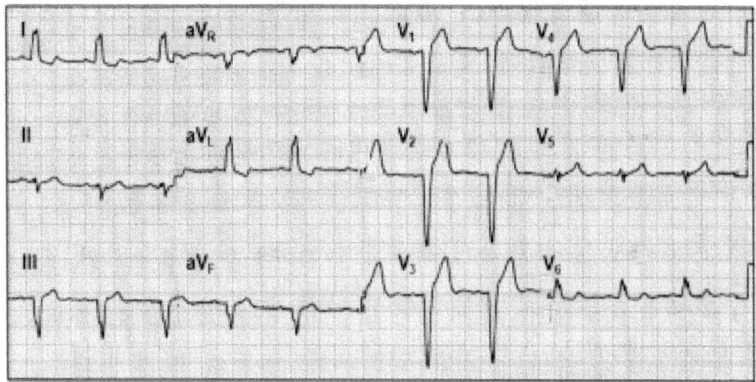

12. Intraventricular Conduction Defect. Your diagnosis?

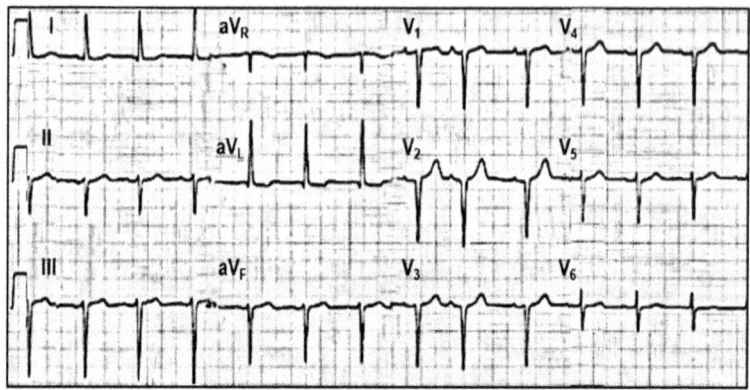

13. Intraventricular Conduction Defect. Your diagnosis?

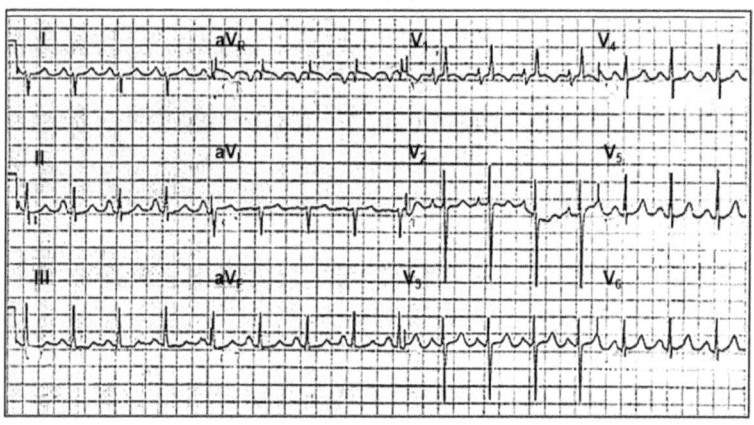

Chapter 6

Coronary Artery Disease

Coronary artery disease (CAD), also known as atherosclerotic heart disease, coronary heart disease, or ischemic heart disease, is a narrowing of one or more of the coronary arteries that supply blood to the heart. These are:

- Left main coronary artery and its branches
  - Circumflex coronary artery
  - Left anterior descending coronary artery
- Right coronary artery

Coronary artery disease is divided into (1) stable angina, (2) unstable angina, (3) non-ST segment elevation myocardial infarction, and (4) ST segment elevation myocardial infarction.

STABLE ANGINA

In an individual with stable angina (SA), attacks occur with predictable frequency and duration and are precipitated by circumstances such as exercise or emotional stress, both of which increase myocardial oxygen demand. Stable angina does not occur at rest.

Stable angina symptoms usually develop when there is greater than 70 percent stenosis of a major coronary artery (left anterior descending, circumflex, or right coronary artery). Multiple tandem stenoses in one artery can at times cause angina, even if a coronary artery is less than 50 percent obstructed. Stenosis of the left main coronary artery can cause symptoms when only 50 percent stenosis is present.

Depression greater than or equal to one millimeter at 0.08 seconds after the end of the QRS complex (J-point) in a limb lead or two millimeters in a precordial lead is considered diagnostic of coronary artery disease.

The three types of ST segment depressions are shown in Figure 6-1. The horizontal ST segment depression is the most predictive of coronary ischemia, with downsloping of the ST segment the next most predictive, followed by slow upsloping of the ST segment, which is the least predictive.

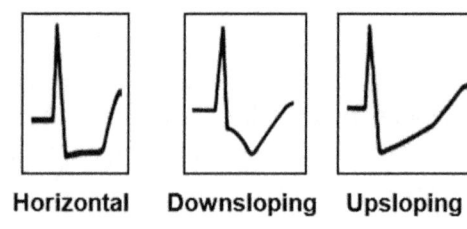

Horizontal   Downsloping   Upsloping

Figure 6-1. Three types of ST segment depressions.

Figure 6-2 shows ST segment depression in the lateral leads of an ECG in a patient who is asymptomatic at rest (stable coronary artery disease) but has angina with activity consisting of downsloping ST segment depressions in the chest leads.

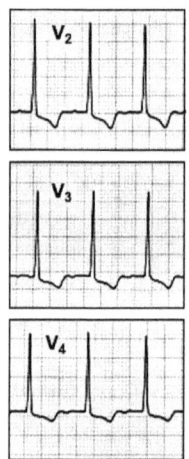

Figure 6-2. Downward sloping of ST segments in leads V₂, V₃, and V₄ of a patient who is asymptomatic at rest, but who has angina and develops these changes with activity.

Not all patients with coronary artery disease show ST segment depressions during periods of chest pain. To assist in the diagnosis of coronary artery disease in these patients, an electrocardiogram is recorded while the patient exercises under controlled conditions (*stress testing*). About 10 percent of normal men will have a false-positive test for angina. False-positive tests are particularly common in women. False-negative tests also occur.

Other conditions to consider in the presence of ST segment depression include:

- Acute posterior myocardial infarction
- Drug effects (digoxin, type 1a antiarrhythmics such as quinidine)
- Electrolyte effects (hypokalemia, hypercalcemia, hypomagnesemia)
- Hypothermia
- Left bundle branch block
- Pulmonary embolus
- Reciprocal changes representing cardiac injury in other leads
- Supraventricular tachycardia
- Ventricular hypertrophy with strain

PRINZMETAL'S ANGINA

Prinzmetal's angina is atypical angina that occurs at rest and results in ST segment elevation, as opposed to the ST segment depression of other forms of angina. The cause is thought to be transient ischemia due to vasospasm. Prinzmetal's angina may occur in individuals with otherwise normal coronary arteries.

The coronary arteries can spasm as a result of:

- Exposure to cold weather
- Stress
- Medications
- Smoking
- Cocaine use

The pain or discomfort of Prinzmetal's angina:

- Usually occurs at rest and during the night or early morning hours
- Is usually severe
- Relieved by medications, such as nitrates and calcium channel blockers

UNSTABLE ANGINA

The three different presentations of *unstable angina (UA)* are:

- Exertional angina of new onset, even if it is relieved by rest and requires a considerable amount of exertion to produce symptoms.
- Exertional angina that was previously stable and now occurs with less physical exertion.
- Anginal symptoms at rest without physical exertion.

The ECG presentation of unstable angina is essentially the same as stable angina, except for the times at which it occurs.

Wellen's Syndrome

Wellen's syndrome is a proximal left anterior descending coronary artery stenosis in patients with unstable angina. The ECG patterns (Figure 6-3) show:

- Symmetric deeply inverted T waves in leads V₂ and V₃ or
- Biphasic T waves in leads V₂ and V₃ (less common)

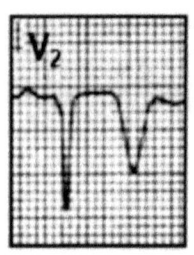

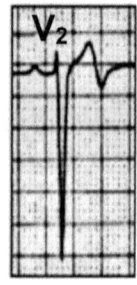

Figure 6-3. The ECG patterns of Wellen's syndrome.

Symmetric deeply inverted T wave

Biphasic T wave

Recognition of the ECG abnormality is important because Wellen's syndrome is a preinfarction stage of coronary artery disease that often progresses to an anterior wall infarction. A stress test should not be done because it can cause infarction; instead, these patients should go to the cath lab.

MYOCARDIAL INFARCTION

Myocardial infarction may occur with ST segment elevation or without ST segment elevation. The ECG is relatively nonspecific for myocardial infarction, missing up to 50 percent of them in the early stages. If a myocardial infarction is suspected and the ECG does not confirm it, the ECG should be repeated after a period of time.

Non-ST Segment Elevation Myocardial Infarction

Non-ST segment elevation myocardial infarction (NSTEMI) also results in anginal symptoms at rest. It is the result of complete occlusion of a minor coronary artery or a partial occlusion of a major coronary artery by atherosclerosis. ST segment elevation does not occur. Some necrosis of cardiac muscle occurs, resulting in elevated biomarkers (myoglobin, troponins, creatine kinase).

- **Myoglobin**: Myoglobin is released into the circulation with damage to skeletal or cardiac muscle tissue. The benefit of myoglobin determination in the absence of a skeletal muscle etiology is the fact that a detectable increase is seen in patients with cardiac symptoms 30 minutes after cardiac muscle damage occurs, unlike the troponins and creatine kinase which can take 3-4 hours to rise.

- **Troponins**: The enzymes troponin I and troponin T are proteins important in the contractile apparatus of cardiac muscle cells. They are released into the circulation about 3-4 hours after myocardial infarction and are detectable for 10 days or so afterwards. Troponin elevations are much more sensitive than myoglobin and CK for myocardial infarction.

- **Creatine kinase (CK)**: Creatine kinase, also known as creatine phosphokinase (CPK), is a muscle enzyme that exists in isoenzyme forms. The MB type (MB-CK) is specific for myocardial cells. The CK-MB level increases approximately 3-4 hours after a myocardial infarction and remains elevated for 3-4 days.

The time course of cardiac biomarkers after a myocardial infarction is shown in figure 6-4.

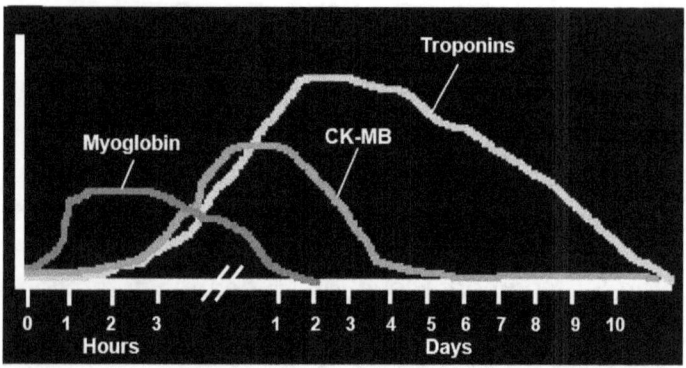

Figure 6-4. Cardiac biomarkers after a myocardial infarction.

Because it is often difficult to tell UA from NSTEMI, the terms together are called non-ST-elevation acute coronary syndrome (NSTE-ACS).

ST Segment Elevation Myocardial Infarction

ST segment elevation myocardial infarction (STEMI) involves anginal symptoms at rest resulting from complete occlusion of a major coronary artery by a thrombus. It results in necrosis of cardiac muscle as identified by elevated cardiac biomarkers and ST segment elevations on the 12-lead electrocardiogram.

STEMI is a life-threatening emergency that must be diagnosed and treated promptly, if possible via coronary revascularization by percutaneous coronary intervention (PCI); that is, placing a stint in the blocked artery. Coronary angiography is done first to see if the patient is a candidate for PCI. If PCI is not available, the obstructing thrombus may be lysed with tissue plasminogen activator (tPA).

The first ECG change during STEMI is hyperacute T waves (tall, narrow, pointed, symmetrical) which are related to localized hyperkalemia (Figure 6-5). These changes are rarely seen by the physician because they are transient and frequently disappear prior to hospital arrival.

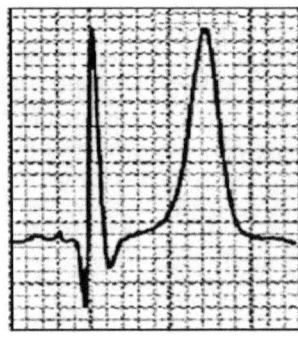

Figure 6-5. Hyperacute T waves of very early STEMI.

The ST segment elevation of STEMI is said to resemble a tombstone, and a patient with this pattern is said to be "Tombstoning" (Figure 6-6). Be sure not to say this in front of the patient, even if you believe he or she is unconscious.

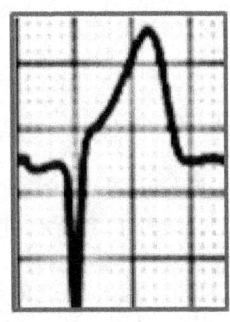 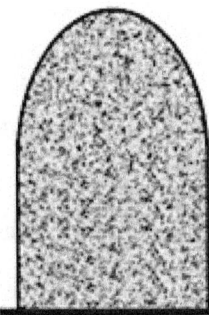

Figure 6-6. Tombstoning.

STEMI is diagnosed electrocardiographically by examining the QRS complexes, ST segments, and T waves. Combinations of abnormalities in various leads are required to make the diagnosis. Changes over time (minutes to hours) may be required to firmly diagnose STEMI.

Figure 6.7 shows the evolution of the QRS complex, ST segment, and T wave from minutes to months after a STEMI. During

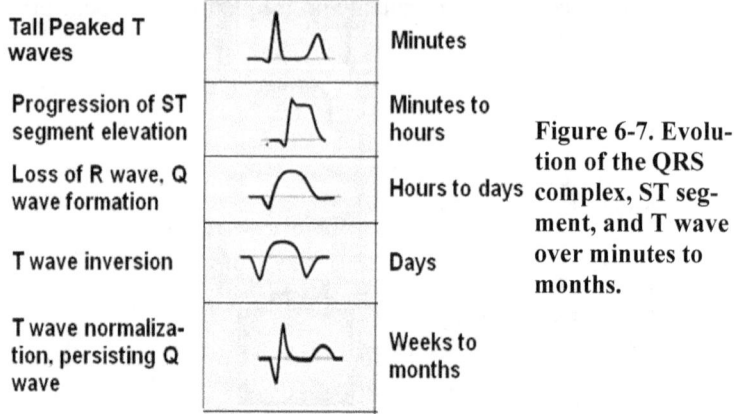

Tall Peaked T waves		Minutes
Progression of ST segment elevation		Minutes to hours
Loss of R wave, Q wave formation		Hours to days
T wave inversion		Days
T wave normalization, persisting Q wave		Weeks to months

Figure 6-7. Evolution of the QRS complex, ST segment, and T wave over minutes to months.

the evolving phase, the ST segments begin returning toward the baseline and the T waves become inverted, eventually returning to their normal positions. In most cases, however, abnormal Q waves persist for months and even years and become the basis for diagnosing an old STEMI.

Anterior STEMI

Anterior STEMI may be divided into:

- **Strictly anterior STEMI**: ST segment elevations in leads V_3 and V_4.
- **Anteroseptal STEMI**: Loss of the normal small septal R waves in leads V_1 and V_2 as well as ST segment elevations in leads V_3-V_4
- **Anterolateral STEMI**: ST segment elevations in the more laterally situated chest leads (V_5-V_6) and the left lateral limb leads (I, aV_L) as well as the anterior leads V_3-V_4.

Criteria for anterior STEMI include:

- New ST elevation at the J point in at least 2 contiguous leads of greater than 2 mm (0.2 mV) in men in leads V_2–V_3
- New ST elevation at the J point in at least 2 contiguous leads of greater than 1.5 mm (0.15 mV) in women in leads V_2–V_3

- And/or ST segment elevation greater than 1 mm (0.1 mV) in other contiguous chest leads or limb leads

The *de Winter ECG pattern* is an anterior STEMI equivalent that presents without obvious ST segment elevation. Instead, the key diagnostic features include upsloping ST depressions and peaked T waves in the precordial leads (Figure 6-8). The de Winter ECG pattern results from occlusion of the LAD coronary artery. It represents an acute process unlike Wellen's sign which represents a subacute process.

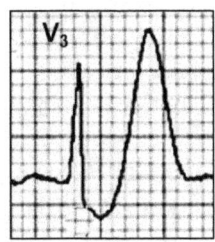

Figure 6-8. De Winter ECG pattern

An anterolateral STEMI is shown in Figure 6-9. Notice the reciprocal depressions in the inferior leads (II, III and aV$_F$).

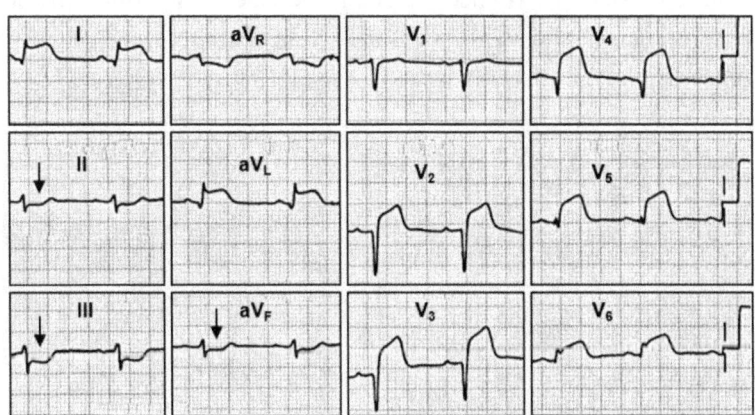

Figure 6-9. Anterolateral STEMI. Note the ST segment elevations in the anterior chest leads and leads I and aVL and the reciprocal ST segment depressions in the inferior leads II, III, and aV$_F$.

Anterior STEMI has the highest mortality rate because it can suddenly cause third degree heart block, ventricular fibrillation, or ventricular tachycardia.

Other conditions to consider in the presence of ST segment elevation include:

- Acute pericarditis
- Myocarditis
- Athletic heart syndrome
- Cardiomyopathy
- CNS events, such as subarachnoid hemorrhage
- Early repolarization
- Hyperkalemia
- Left ventricular aneurysm
- Reciprocal changes due to ischemia in other leads
- Vasospasm due to cocaine or methamphetamine abuse

Anterior infarction interrupts the normal R wave progression in the chest leads, so R wave progression should be noted when reading an electrocardiogram (Figure 6-10).

To check for normal R wave progression, first look at lead V_1; it should have a small R wave. Next look at lead V_6; it should have a large R wave. Next check to see if the isoelectric point falls between leads V_3 and V_4. If all of these things are true, then R wave progression is most likely normal.

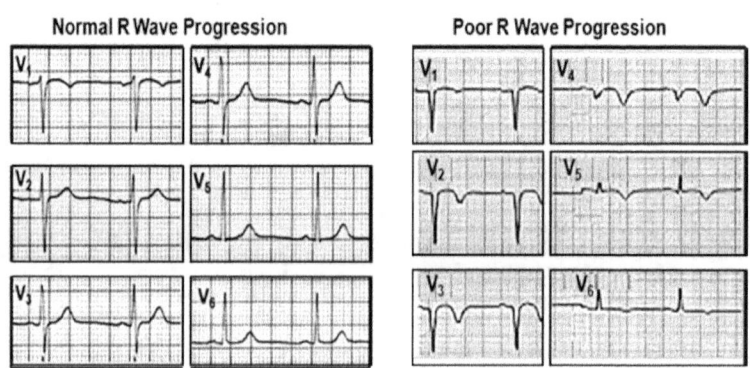

Figure 6-10. Normal R wave progression (left) and poor R wave progression (right).

Poor R wave progression is not specific for anterior myocardial infarction. Other conditions to consider in the presence of poor R wave progression include:

- Cardiomyopathy
- Chest wall deformity
- Complete or incomplete LBBB
- Diffuse infiltrative cardiac disease
- Lead misplacement
- Left anterior fascicular block
- Left anterior hemiblock
- Normal variant
- Pulmonary disease (COPD, chronic asthma)
- Ventricular hypertrophy (LVH, RVH)
- Wolff-Parkinson-White syndrome

Inferior STEMI

Inferior STEMI involves the diaphragmatic portion of the left ventricle and is indicated by:

- ST segment elevations in leads that explore the heart from below (II, III, aV$_F$).
- Reciprocal ST segment depression in the lateral leads (I, aV$_L$,V$_5$-V$_6$)

An electrocardiogram tracing from a patient with an inferior STEMI is shown in Figure 6-11.

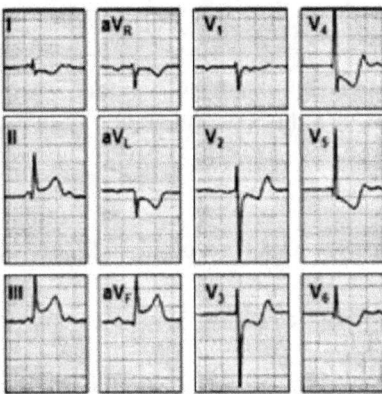

Figure 6-11. Electrocardiogram tracing typical of an inferior STEMI. Note the ST segment elevations in leads II, III, and aV$_F$ and the reciprocal ST segment depressions in the lateral chest leads.

Right ventricular infarction complicates up to 40% of inferior STEMIs. Isolated RV infarction is extremely uncommon.

Patients with RV infarction are very preload sensitive and can develop severe hypotension in response to nitrates or other preload-reducing agents. Hypotension in right ventricular infarction is treated with I.V. fluids.

In patients presenting with an inferior STEMI, right ventricular infarction is suggested by:

- ST elevation in V_1 (the only standard ECG lead that looks directly at the right ventricle).
- ST elevation in lead III > lead II (lead III is more rightward facing than lead II and hence more sensitive to the injury current produced by the right ventricle.

An ECG of a patient with an inferior STEMI and right ventricular infarction is shown in figure 6-12.

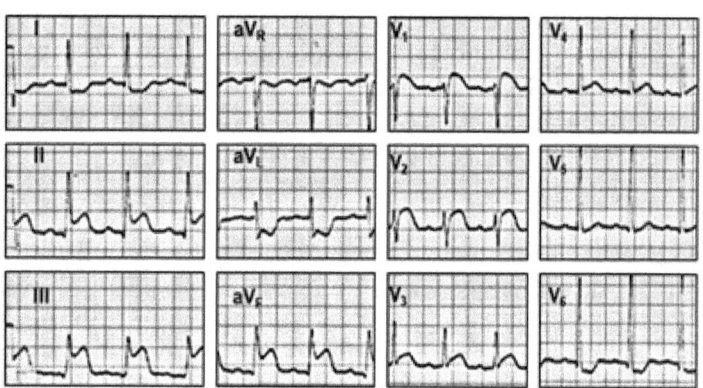

Figure 6-12. Inferior STEMI with right ventricular infarct. Note the ST segment elevation in lead V_1 and the ST segment elevation in lead III greater than in lead II.

Inferior STEMI may be associated with bradycardia and hypotension. Nausea may be present. A Mobitz type I block may occur.

Posterior STEMI

Posterior infarction involves the posterior wall of the left ventricle.

It does not generate Q wave formation or ST segment elevation in the conventional 12-lead electrocardiogram because there are no posterior exploring electrodes. Instead, the ECG changes of posterior infarction are seen as reciprocal changes; that is, they are seen upside down in the leads monitoring the anterior part of the heart. Q waves are seen as R waves, ST elevations are seen as depressions, and T wave inversions are seen as an upright T waves. Posterior STEMI can be documented with the use of additional posterior leads.

The ECG findings of an acute posterior wall infarction include:

- The ratio of the R wave to the S wave in leads V_1 or V_2 is > 1.
- ST segment depression in the septal and precordial leads (V_1 to V_4).
- ST elevation in additional posterior leads to the normal 12-lead ECG (leads V_{4R}, V_8, V_9) when used.
- Unlike right ventricular hypertrophy with R/S is greater than 1 in lead V_1 or V_2, right axis deviation is not present with posterior infarction.
- Inferior infarction sometimes occurs with posterior infarction. In this case, ST segment elevations in the inferior leads (II, III, and aV_F) would also be present.

The ECG of a patient with a posterior STEMI is shown in figure 6-13.

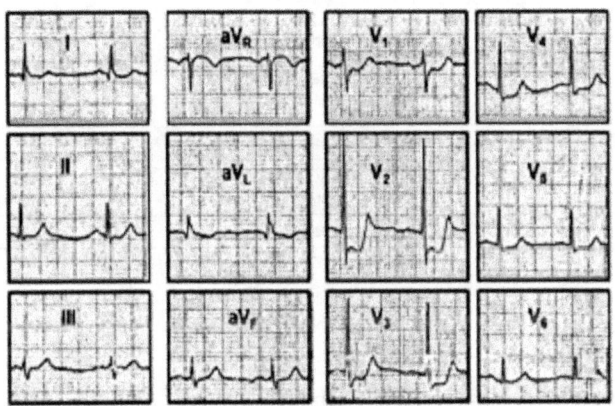

Figure 6-13. Electrocardiogram typical of a posterior STEMI. Note the R > S in lead V_2, the ST depressions in the chest leads, and the absence of right axis deviation

Other conditions to consider in the presence of tall R waves in leads V_1 or V_2 include:

- Dextrocardia (rare)
- Duchenne muscular dystrophy (rare)
- Right bundle branch block
- Right ventricular hypertrophy
- Some normal children and young adults
- Wolff-Parkinson-White syndrome

Myocardial Infarction, ECG Leads, and Involved Coronary Arteries

Table 6-1 shows the relationship among myocardial infarction location, ECG leads affected, and the coronary arteries involved.

Localization	ST Elevation	Reciprocal ST Depression	Coronary Artery
Anterior MI	Leads V_3-V_4	None	Left
Anteroseptal MI	Leads V_1-V_4, disappearance of septal Q waves in leads V_1 & V_2	none	Left
Anterolateral MI	Leads I, aVL, V_3-V_6	Leads II,III, aV$_F$	Left
Septal MI	Leads V_1-V_2, disappearance of septal Q waves in leads V_1 & V_2	None	Left
Inferior MI	Leads II, III, aV$_F$	Leads I, aV$_L$	Right (80%) or circumflex (20%)
Lateral MI	Leads I, aVL, V_5-V_6	Leads II, III, aVF	Left and/or Right
Posterior MI	none	Tall R in leads V_1-V_3 with ST depression in leads V_1-V_3 > 2mm	Right or circumflex
Right Ventricle MI	Lead V_1	Leads I, aV$_L$	Right

OLD STEMI

Old STEMIs are diagnosed by the presence of diagnostic Q waves. Figure 6-14 shows an inferior STEMI a year or so after the initial event. Note the diagnostic Q waves in leads II, III, and aV$_F$.

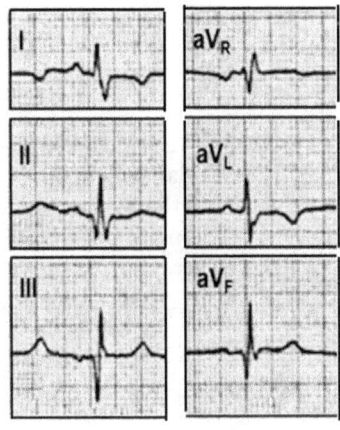

Figure 6-14. Old inferior STEMI. Note the Q waves in leads II, III, and aV_F

For a Q wave to be significant its duration must be at least 0.04 seconds and its amplitude must be at least 25 percent of the amplitude of the following R wave. If both criteria are not met, the Q wave is considered to be non-diagnostic. For instance, small septal Q waves in the lateral leads (V_5-V_6) result from depolarization of the septum and are a normal occurrence. Also, a small Q wave may be present in lead III, which is a normal finding.

Q waves representing various old infarction locations are leads II, III, and aV_F for inferior infarction; leads I, AV_L, and V_5-V_6 for lateral infarction; and leads V_3-V_4 for anterior infarction.

LEFT VENTRICULAR ANEURYSM

Following an acute STEMI, the ST segments usually return towards baseline over a period of about two weeks, while the Q waves persist. However, some degree of ST segment elevation may remain, the result of a left ventricular aneurysm from transmural scarring (Figure 6-15).

The ECG picture of a ventricular aneurysm consists of:

- ST segment elevation two weeks after an acute myocardial infarction.
- Usually associated with well-formed Q waves or QS waves
- Most commonly seen in the precordial leads.
- T waves have a relatively small amplitude in comparison to the QRS complex, unlike the hyperacute T waves of an acute STEMI.

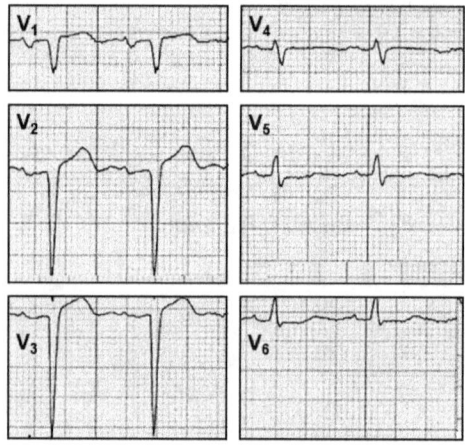

Figure 6-15. Left ventricular aneurysm. Note the ST segment elevations and the QS waves.

Factors favoring ventricular aneurysm over STEMI include:

- Absence of reciprocal ST segment depressions
- Well-formed Q waves
- No symptoms of acute STEMI

SILENT MYOCARDIAL INFARCTION

A silent myocardial infarction is one that produces none of the characteristic symptoms and signs of myocardial infarction. It is thought to occur with significant frequency in diabetics, although there is some question about this. Typical ECG changes would be present acutely if one were to obtain an ECG for some other reason.

STEMI AND BUNDLE BRANCH BLOCKS

STEMI and Left Bundle Branch Block

Traditionally it was taught that acute myocardial infarction could not be diagnosed in the presence of a left bundle branch block (LBBB); however, Sgarbossa et al in 1996 devised a point scoring system to aid in the diagnosis. This is called the Sgarbossa criteria and consists of:

- ST elevation > 1 mm and in the same direction (concordant) as the QRS complex (5 points).
- ST depression > 1 mm in leads V_1, V_2, or V_3 (3 points)
- ST elevation > 5 mm and in the opposite direction (discordant) with the QRS complex (2 points)

A score of at least 3 points is required to suggest an acute STEMI. The criteria are illustrated in Figure 6-16. Sgarbossa criteria are 90% specificity of a STEMI with a sensitivity of 36%).

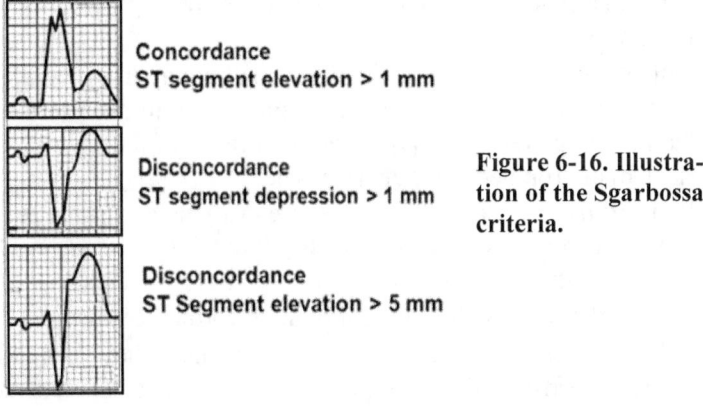

Concordance
ST segment elevation > 1 mm

Disconcordance
ST segment depression > 1 mm

Disconcordance
ST Segment elevation > 5 mm

Figure 6-16. Illustration of the Sgarbossa criteria.

The presence of a new LBBB on the ECG of a patient with chest pain indicates an acute STEMI until proven otherwise.

STEMI and Right Bundle Branch Block

Generally speaking, because RBBB does not affect the left ventricle significantly, RBBB does not mimic or obscure the ECG diagnosis of acute STEMI the way LBBB does.

PSEUDOINFARCTION SYNDROMES

Several pathological conditions may present electrocardiographic findings similar to those of myocardial infarction. They are called *pseudoinfarction syndromes*.

Pseudoinfarction syndromes include:

- Complete or incomplete LBBB may show QS waves or poor R wave progression in leads V_1–V_3.
- Dramatic alterations of ST segments and T waves may occur with increased intracranial pressure due to changes in repolarization that result from enhanced sympathetic nervous system activity.
- Hyperkalemia may show ST segment elevation and peaked T waves.
- LAH may show small Q waves in the anterior chest leads
- Left ventricular aneurysm after extensive infarction may show persistent ST segment elevations
- LVH may show a QS pattern or poor R wave progression in leads V_1-V_3
- Patients with hypertrophic cardiomyopathy may have significant Q waves on their electrocardiograms due to distortion of the normal pattern of depolarization because of the asymmetrical, hypertrophied ventricular muscle.
- Pericarditis may show ST segment elevations and subsequent T wave inversions; however, with pericarditis there is no Q wave formation.
- Pneumothorax may show loss of right precordial R waves
- Pulmonary emphysema and cor pulmonale may show loss of R waves in leads V_1-V_3 and/or inferior Q waves and right axis deviation
- RVH may show tall R waves in leads V_1 or V_2 mimicking true posterior myocardial infarction.

ATHLETIC HEART SYNDROME

Although *athletic heart syndrome* is a benign condition a variety of abnormal ECG patterns occur in 40 percent of athletes. A small subgroup of these shows striking ECG abnormalities that suggest cardiovascular disease. However, these changes are an innocent consequence of long-term, intense athletic training. The majority of these findings are related to increased vagal tone.

The ECG findings in athletic heart syndrome may include:

- Resting sinus bradycardia is the most frequent abnormal

finding in ECGs of well-conditioned athletes. Marathon runners may have heart rates as low as 35 bpm.

- Athletes also have a considerably higher incidence of first and second-degree atrioventricular block, more premature atrial beats, and slightly more premature ventricular beats.
- Increased QRS complex height may be present, giving the appearance of left or right ventricular hypertrophy.
- Widened QRS complexes may simulate incomplete right bundle branch block.
- Repolarization changes may include ST segment elevation indicative of early repolarization.
- Flipped T waves may occur.

A typical ECG of a well-trained athlete is shown is Figure 6-17.

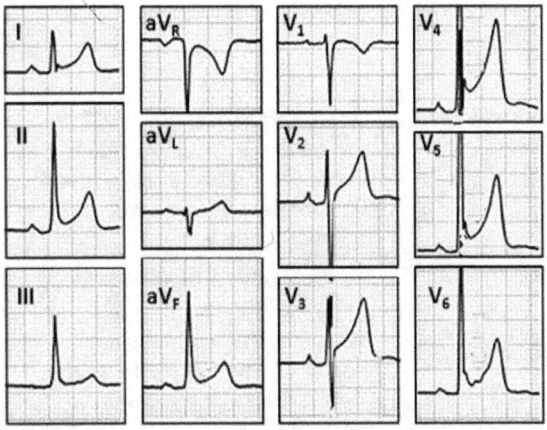

Figure 6-17. ECG from a well-trained athlete showing athletic heart syndrome. Note the early repolarization, left ventricular hypertrophy, and peaked T waves. Sinus bradycardia also was present.

Chapter 6 Quiz

1. The pain of Prinzmetal's angina
   A. Involves stenosed coronary arteries
   B. Usually occurs during the daytime
   C. Is usually mild
   D. Can be relieved by taking medications, such as calcium channel blockers

2. If you are unsure whether a patient has Wellen's syndrome or not you should order an exercise stress test to make the determination (T or F).

Match

3. Strictly anterior STEMI	**A.** ST segment elevations in the more laterally situated chest leads (V_5-V_6) and the left lateral limb leads (I, aV_L) as well as the anterior leads V_3 - V_4.
4. Anteroseptal STEMI	**B.** ST segment elevations in leads V_3 and V_4.
5. Anterolateral STEMI:	**C.** Loss of the normal small septal R waves in leads V_1 and V_2 and ST segment elevations in leads V_3-V_4

Match

6. Inferior STEMI	**A.** ST elevation in lead V_1 and ST segment elevation in lead III > lead II
7. Right ventricular infarction with inferior STEMI	**B.** The ratio of the R wave to the S wave in leads V_1 or V_2 is > 1 without RAD
8. Posterior STEMI	**C.** ST segment elevaton in leads II, III, and aVF

Some ECGs to interpret. Use the 8 steps discussed in Chapter 1.

9.

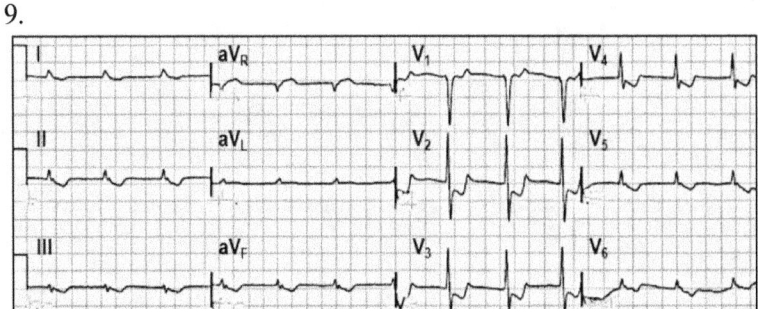

10.

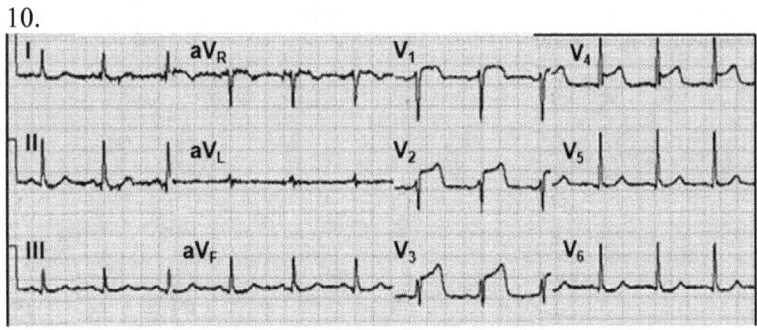

11.

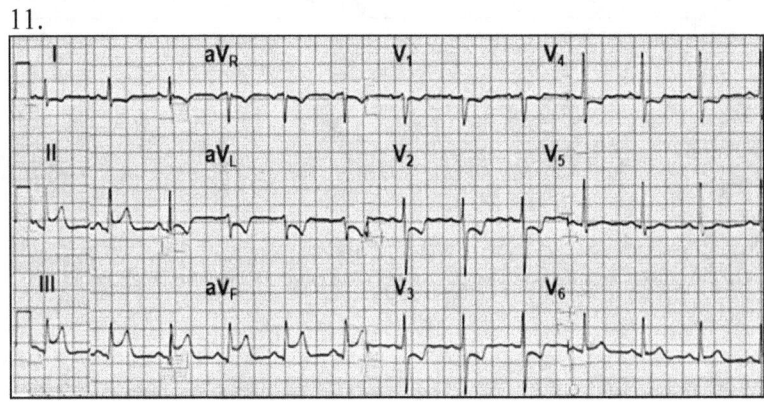

12. No symptoms and cardiac markers not elevated

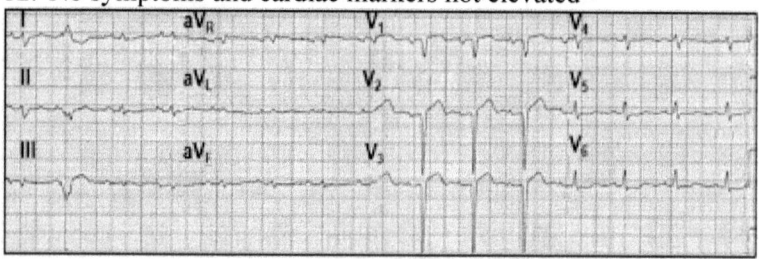

13.

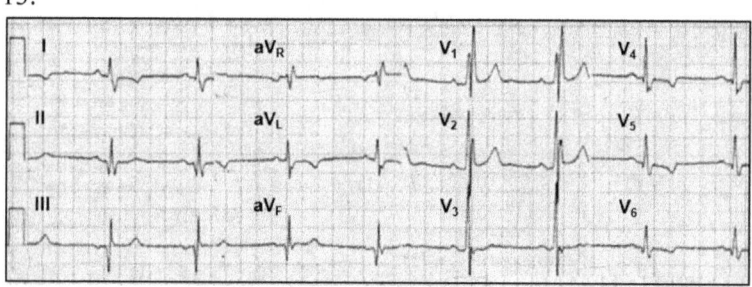

14.

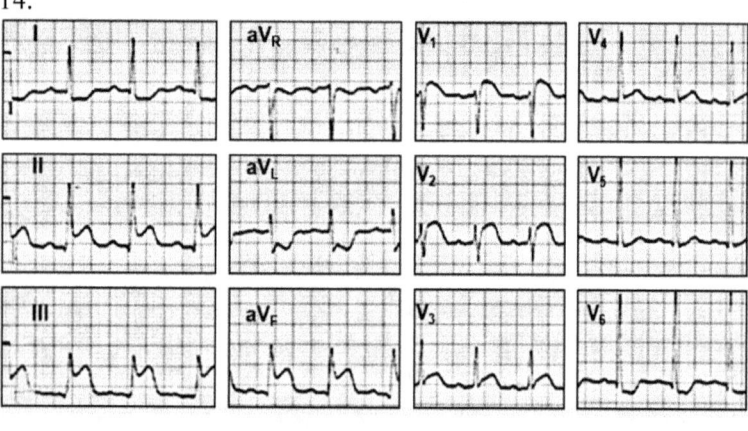

15.

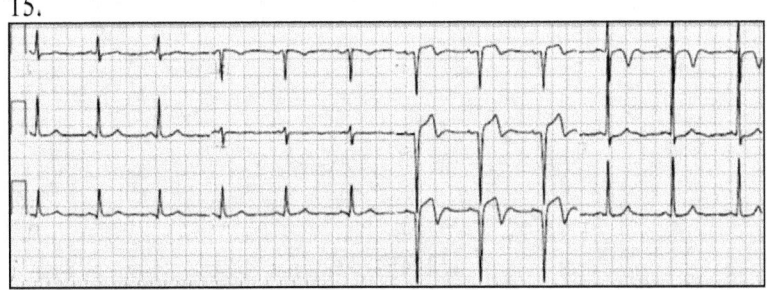

Chapter 7

Rhythm Disturbances

Rhythm disturbances may originate in the sinoatrial node, the atria, the atrioventricular node, the atrioventricular junction, and the ventricles. They can be categorized as:

- **Regular.** RR interval constant (except for minor variation with respiration)
- **Regularly irregular.** RR interval variable, but with a definite pattern (normal beats and ectopic beats grouped together and the grouping repeating over and over)
- **Irregularly irregular.** RR interval variable with no pattern (totally irregular)

Examples or the types of rhythm disturbances are given in Figure 7-1.

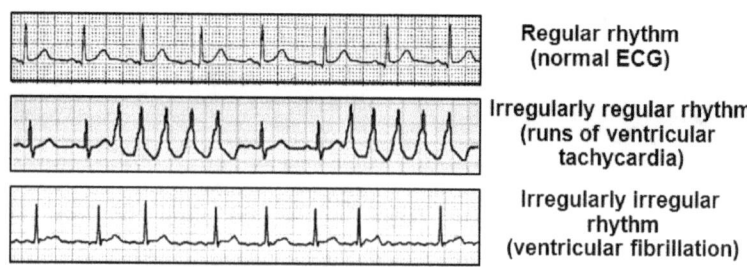

Regular rhythm
(normal ECG)

Irregularly regular rhythm
(runs of ventricular
tachycardia)

Irregularly irregular
rhythm
(ventricular fibrillation)

Figure 7-1. Examples of regular, irregularly regular, and irregularly irregular rhythms.

SINUS RHYTHMS

Sinus rhythms originate in the *sinoatrial node*. Diagnosing sinus rhythms requires examining leads II and aV$_R$ for the correct polarity of the P waves. The P wave is normally positive in lead II and negative in lead aV$_R$. A P wave should precede each QRS complex and the PR interval should be relatively constant.

Normal Sinus Rhythm

Normal sinus rhythm (NSR) is defined as a sinus rhythm with a heart rate between 60 and 100 bpm (Figure 7-2). The rate may vary slightly in a phasic manner due to breathing, increasing with inhalation and decreasing with exhalation. It should not vary by more than 10 percent.

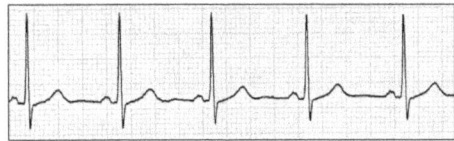

Figure 7-2. Normal sinus rhythm with a rate of about 75 bpm.

Sinus Tachycardia

Sinus tachycardia is a sinus rhythm with a heart rate greater than 100 bpm (Figure 7-3). With sinus tachycardia at very fast rates, the P waves may merge with the preceding T waves and be indistinct. For this reason, tachycardia originating above the ventricles (sinoatrial node, atrial muscle, atrioventricular junction) is often referred to as *supraventricular tachycardia (SVT)* without specifying its site of origin.

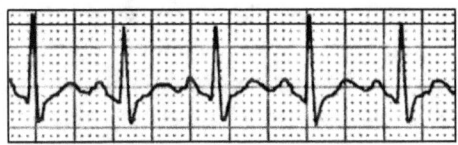

Figure 7-3. Sinus tachycardia with a rate of about 130 bpm

Sinus tachycardia occurs for many reasons, including:

- Anxiety
- Congestive heart failure
- Hyperthyroidism
- Hypotension
- Physical activity
- Sympathomimetic drugs

Sinus Bradycardia

Sinus bradycardia is a sinus rhythm with a heart rate less than 60 bpm (Figure 7-4).

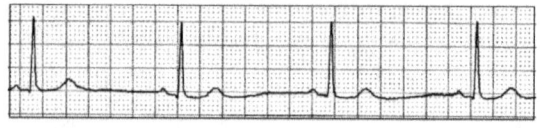

Figure 7-4. Sinus bradycardia with a rate of 45bpm.

Sinus bradycardia occurs for many reasons, including:

- Drugs that increase vagal tone (digoxin)
- Drugs that decrease sympathetic tone (beta blockers)
- Hypothyroidism
- Physical conditioning. World-class marathon runners may have resting heart rates as low as 35 bpm.

Sinoatrial Block

Sinoatrial block refers to failure of the sinus node to function for one or more beats. In this condition there is one or more missing beats; that is, no P waves or QRS complexes are seen (Figure 7-5). Fortunately, when the sinus fails to function for a significant period of time (*sinus arrest*), another part of the conduction system usually assumes the role of pacemaker. These pacing beats are referred to as *escape beats* and may come from the atrial muscle, the atrioventricular junction, or the ventricles. When the sinoatrial node fails to function and another area of the heart does not take over the pacemaker role, *asystole* occurs and the electrocardiogram shows a straight-line pattern.

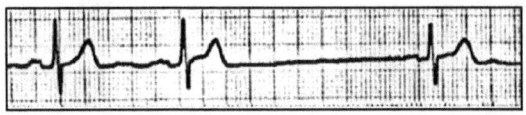

Figure 7-5. Sinoatrial block. Note the missing P wave and QRS complex.

Sinoatrial block can occur for a variety of reasons, including:

- Ischemia
- Inflammation
- Infiltrative process
- Fibrotic disease
- Excessive vagal tone
- Drugs (digoxin, procainamide, quinidine)

Sick Sinus Syndrome

In elderly people the sinus node may undergo degenerative changes and fail to function effectively. Periods of sinus arrest, sinus tachycardia, and sinus bradycardia may occur, leading to episodes of lightheadedness or even syncope. This has been termed *sick sinus syndrome* (Figure 7-6). Treatment of symptomatic individuals may require a permanent pacemaker to control the periods of bradycardia. This may be combined with drugs such as digoxin or a beta-blocker to control the periods of tachycardia.

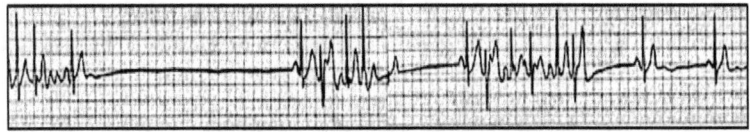

Figure 7-6. Sick sinus syndrome.

NON-SINUS ATRIAL ARRHYTHMIAS

Non-sinus atrial arrhythmias include premature atrial beats, paroxysmal atrial tachycardia, multifocal atrial tachycardia, atrial flutter, and atrial fibrillation. Because the stimuli arise above the level of the ventricles, the QRS pattern is usually normal.

Premature Atrial Contraction

A *premature atrial contraction (PAC)* is an ectopic beat arising from somewhere in either atrium, but not in the sinoatrial node. Premature atrial contractions occur before the next expected normal beat, and a slight pause usually follows the contraction (Figure 7-7).

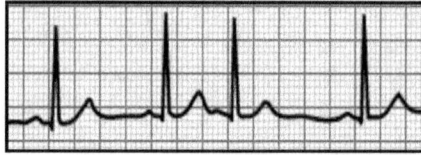

Figure 7-7. Premature atrial contraction. Note the pause following the PAC.

The P wave of the premature beat may have a configuration different than the normal P wave. It may even be of opposite polarity if it arises low in the atria, causing the atrial depolarization wave to travel backwards toward the sinoatrial node. Occasionally the P wave will not be seen because it is lost in the preceding T wave. The PR interval of the premature atrial contraction may be shorter than the normal PR interval.

If the premature atrial depolarization wave reaches the atrioventricular node before the node has had time to repolarize, the impulse may not be conducted. In this case, a premature, abnormal P wave will be seen without a subsequent QRS complex.

Premature atrial beats are sometimes conducted to ventricular tissue during the process of ventricular repolarization. In such cases, the subsequent ventricular depolarization may take place by an abnormal pathway, generating a wide, bizarre QRS complex. This is referred to as *aberrant ventricular depolarization* and is discussed later in this chapter.

Paroxysmal Atrial Tachycardia

Paroxysmal atrial tachycardia (PAT) is defined as three or more consecutive premature atrial contractions in a row. In some cases, the run of paroxysmal atrial tachycardia may be brief and self-limited. In other cases, it may be sustained for hours or even days and require termination by intervention. Paroxysmal atrial tachycardia occurs at a regular rate, usually between 150 and 250 bpm (Figure 7-8).

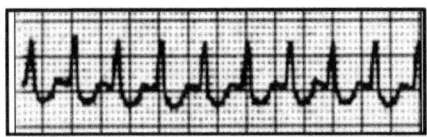

Figure 7-8. Paroxysmal atrial tachycardia with a rate of about 225 bpm.

As with sinus tachycardia, P waves may or may not be seen, and it may be difficult to differentiate paroxysmal atrial tachycardia from sinus tachycardia. Paroxysmal atrial tachycardia may occur in normal individuals as well as in those with organic heart disease.

Multifocal Atrial Tachycardia

Multifocal atrial tachycardia (MFAT) results from the presence of multiple, different atrial pacemaker foci. This rhythm disturbance is characterized by a tachycardia with beat-to-beat variations of the P wave morphology (Figure 7-9). Multifocal atrial tachycardia most commonly occurs in individuals with chronic pulmonary disease.

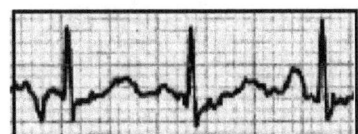

Figure 7-9. Multifocal atrial tachycardia. Note the varying P wave morphology.

Atrial Flutter

Atrial flutter is also an ectopic atrial rhythm. Instead of P waves, characteristic sawtooth waves are seen. The atrial rate in atrial flutter is usually about 300 bpm. However, the atrioventricular junction is unable to conduct at this rapid rate so the ventricular rate is less—usually 150 bpm, 100 bpm, 75 bpm, and so on.

Atrial flutter with a ventricular rate of 150 bpm is called two-to-one flutter because of the ratio of the atrial rate to the ventricular rate (300 bpm/150 bpm = 2/1); a ventricular rate of 100 bpm is three-to-one flutter (300 bpm/100 bpm = 3/1), and a ventricular rate of 75 bpm is a four-to-one flutter (300 bpm/75 bpm = 4/1). The ventricular rate may abruptly change from one rate to another as the degree of block at the atrioventricular junction changes.

The sawtooth pattern of atrial flutter is best seen in the inferior leads (II, III, aV_F). An example of atrial flutter is shown in Figure 7-10. Although atrial flutter is not specific for any particular type of heart disease, it is rarely seen in individuals with normal hearts.

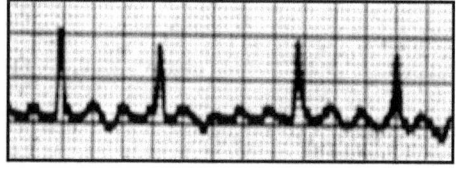

Figure 7-10. Atrial flutter with abrupt change from 2:1 flutter to 4:1 and back again.

Atrial flutter can occur with:

- Alcohol abuse
- COPD
- Mitral valve disease
- Myocardial infarction
- Pulmonary embolism
- Thyrotoxicosis

Atrial Fibrillation

In *atrial fibrillation (AF)* the atria are depolarized at an extremely rapid rate, greater than 400 bpm. This fibrillatory activity produces a characteristic irregular, wavy base-line pattern instead of normal P waves. The baseline pattern may be classified as coarse or fine.

Because the atrioventricular junction is refractory to most of the impulses reaching it, it allows only a fraction of them to pass through to the ventricles. The ventricular rate is, therefore, only 110 to 180 bpm.

Also characteristic of atrial fibrillation is a haphazardly irregular ventricular rhythm that results from the random stimulation of the atrioventricular junction (variable RR intervals). An example of atrial fibrillation is shown in Figure 7-11.

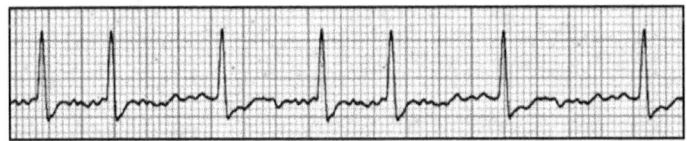

Figure 7-11. Atrial fibrillation. Note the variable RR intervals and lack of P waves.

Atrial fibrillation may occur paroxysmally, lasting only a few minutes, hours, or days, or it may be chronic and persist for years. Atrial fibrillation may occur in normal individuals and in patients with a variety of cardiac diseases. Common causes of atrial fibrillation are:

- Acute alcohol intoxication (holiday heart, Saturday night heart)
- Acute pulmonary processes
- Congestive heart failure
- Coronary artery disease
- Hypertensive heart disease
- Hyperthyroidism
- Narcotic abuse
- Valvular heart disease

JUNCTIONAL RHYTHMS

Junctional rhythms arise in the atrioventricular junction. P waves, when seen, are opposite their normal polarity; that is, negative in lead II and positive in lead aV_R. These are called *retrograde P waves* because they result from the atrial depolarization wave traveling backward from the atrioventricular junction through the atria toward the sinoatrial node. Retrograde P waves may precede, be buried in, or follow the QRS complex. Since the stimulus arises above the level of the ventricles, the QRS complex is usually of normal configuration.

Premature Junctional Contractions

Since the atrioventricular junction also may serve as an ectopic pacemaker, premature junctional beats can occur. *Premature junctional contractions* are similar to premature atrial contractions in that they occur before the next beat is due and a slight pause follows the premature beat (Figure 7-12).

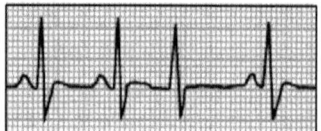

Figure 7-12. Premature junctional contraction. Note the absence of a P wave and the pause after the premature beat.

Junctional Tachycardia

Atrioventricular *junctional tachycardia* is simply a run of three or more premature junctional beats (Figure 7-13). Junctional tachycardia has about the same rate as paroxysmal atrial tachycardia and often cannot be distinguished from it. The difference is not clinically significant.

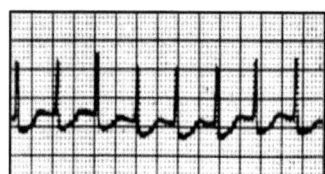

Figure 7-13. Junctional tachycardia at a rate of about 150 bpm.

Junctional Escape Rhythm

An atrioventricular *junctional escape beat* is an escape beat that occurs after a pause in the normal sinus rhythm. Atrial pacing usually resumes after the junctional beat. A *junctional escape rhythm*, defined as a consecutive run of three or more atrioventricular junctional beats, may develop if the sinoatrial node does not resume the pacemaker role. Junctional escape rhythm has a rate between 40 and 60 bpm (Figure 7-14).

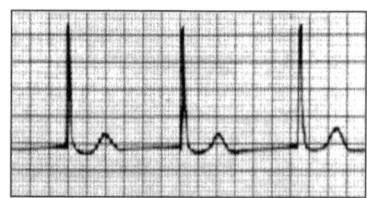

Figure 7-14. Junctional escape rhythm at a rate of 50 bpm.

Atrioventricular junctional escape rhythms may be due to:

- Acute myocardial infarction
- Digoxin toxicity
- Hyperkalemia
- Hypoxia

ATRIOVENTRICULAR HEART BLOCK

Atrioventricular heart block occurs in three forms—first-degree, second-degree, and third-degree. Second-degree heart block is divided into two types—Mobitz type 1 and Mobitz type 2.

There are numerous causes of heart block, and many factors can produce any of the three degrees. Some of these causes are:

- Acute myocardial infarction, particularly inferior infarctions (blood supply to the inferior ventricular wall and the atrioventricular junction arises from the same source)
- Digoxin
- Ischemic heart disease

First-degree Heart Block

The electrocardiographic abnormality of *first-degree heart block* is a prolonged PR interval to greater than 0.2 seconds (Figure 7-15). In addition to the factors already mentioned, hyperkalemia may cause first-degree heart block. First-degree heart block also may be present in normal individuals.

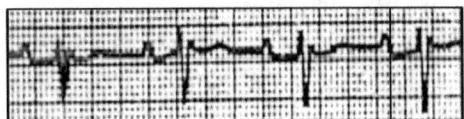

Figure 7-15. First-degree atrioventricular block. Note the prolonged PR interval.

Second-degree Heart Block

There are two types of second-degree atrioventricular block—Mobitz type 1 and Mobitz type 2. When the PR interval becomes progressively longer until a QRS complex is dropped and then the process repeats, this is a second-degree atrioventricular block known as *Mobitz* type 1 block or *Wenckebach* phenomenon (Figure 7-16).

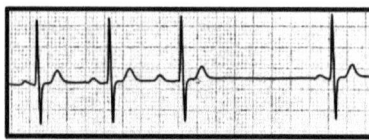

Figure 7-16. Second-degree AV block, Mobitz type 1. Note the progressively increasing PR interval until a QRS complex is dropped.

If the QRS complex is periodically dropped without lengthening of the PR interval, this is called a *Mobitz type 2 block*. A dropped beat is seen as a P wave that is not followed by a QRS complex. Mobitz type 2 heart block is a more severe form of second-degree block because it often progresses to complete heart block.

The characteristic electrocardiogram picture of Mobitz type 2 heart block is that of a series of non-conducted P waves. For example, with a two-to-one block every other P wave is conducted, with a three-to-one block every third P wave is conducted, and with a four-to-one block every fourth P wave is conducted.

An example of Mobitz type 2 block is shown in Figure 7-17.

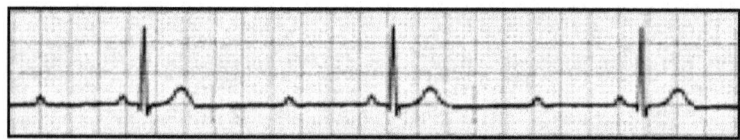

Figure 7-17. Second-degree A-V block, Mobitz type 2. Note the P waves that are not followed by QRS complexes

Third-degree Heart Block

Third-degree heart block is also referred to as *complete heart block* because the atrioventricular junction does not conduct any stimuli from the atria to the ventricles. Instead, the atria and ventricles are paced independently. The characteristic electrocardiogram picture of complete heart block is:

- P waves are present and occur at a faster rate than the ventricular rate.
- QRS complexes are present and occur at a regular rate, usually less than 60 bpm.
- The P waves bear no relationship to the QRS complexes. Thus, the PR intervals are completely variable.

With third-degree heart block, the QRS complex may be of normal or abnormal width, depending on the location of the blockage in the atrioventricular junction. If the blockage is in the first part of the junction (atrioventricular node), the QRS complex will be of normal width. If the blockage is lower in the junction (bundle of His), the ventricles will be paced by an idioventricular pacemaker and the QRS complexes will be abnormally wide. Examples of third-degree heart block are shown in Figure 7-18.

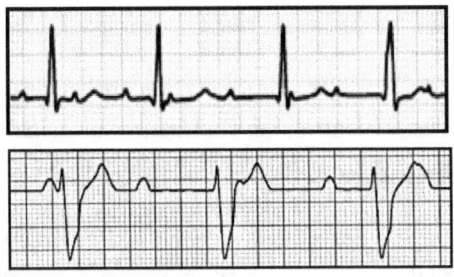

Figure 7-18. Third-degree heart block. (A) Block in the AV node and (B) Block lower in the bundle of His. Note the atria and ventricles beating at separate rates.

Complete heart block also can occur from blockage of the right bundle branch and both fascicles of the left bundle branch.

Complete heart block is usually seen in older individuals who have degenerative changes in their conduction systems. Fainting attacks from complete heart block is known as *Stokes-Adams syndrome*. Seizures sometimes occur.

VENTRICULAR RHYTHM DISTURBANCES

Ventricular tissue also is capable of spontaneous depolarization. Because the depolarization wave arises in the myocardium, it does not follow the normal path of ventricular depolarization. Therefore, the QRS complex is prolonged and bizarre in shape.

In addition to premature ventricular contractions, ectopic

ventricular beats produce ventricular tachycardia and sometimes ventricular fibrillation. Ventricular escape rhythms also occur.

Premature Ventricular Contractions

Premature ventricular contractions (PVCs) are premature beats arising in the ventricles. They are analogous to premature atrial contractions and premature junctional contractions. Premature ventricular contractions have the following characteristics:

- They are premature and arise before the next normal beat is expected (a P wave is not seen before a premature ventricular contraction).
- They are aberrant in appearance. The QRS complex is always abnormally wide, usually greater than 0.12 seconds.
- The T waves and the QRS complexes usually point in the opposite direction.

As with a premature atrial contraction or a premature junctional contraction, a premature ventricular contraction is usually followed by a compensatory pause before the supraventricular mechanism resumes control.

PVCs may be unifocal or multifocal. *Unifocal PVCs* arise from the same ventricular site and, as a result, have the same appearance in a given electrocardiogram. *Multifocal PVCs*, on the other hand, arise from different ventricular foci and have different QRS patterns. Multifocal PVCs are shown in Figure 7-19.

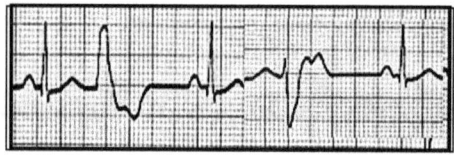

Figure 7-19. Biphasic Premature ventricular contractions. Note the pause after each PVC.

PVCs may occur singularly, as paroxysmal bursts, or be persistent as ventricular tachycardia (V-tach).

PVCs can be seen with virtually any kind of heart disease, particularly after an acute myocardial infarction.

Benign PVCs are common to all age groups, and most often

are due to anxiety or excessive caffeine use. PVCs that occur during exercise are abnormal and their cause should be investigated.

Other causes of PVCs include:

- Cardiac (ischemic heart disease, cardiomyopathy, valvular heart disease, mitral valve prolapse)
- Stimulants (caffeine, cocaine, ephedrine, or pseudoephedrine)
- Alcohol
- Electrolyte abnormalities (hyperkalemia, hypokalemia, hypo-magnesemia)
- Metabolic acidosis
- Hypoxemia
- Medications (digoxin, antipsychotics, tricyclic antidepres-sants)
- Antiarrhythmics (flecainide, sotalol, quinidine)

Supraventricular Beat with Aberrancy

There are two possible etiologies for a wide and premature ventricular depolarization. The first etiology, premature ventricular contraction, has already been discussed. The second etiology is referred to as *aberrant ventricular depolarization.* In this instance, the depolarization wave is initiated above the ventricular level and because it is premature it reaches the ventricles when they are still in a partially depolarized state. This results in a wide QRS complex. The following rules can be used to help differentiate aberrant ventricular depolarization from premature ventricular contraction:

- The beat is aberrant if a P wave precedes the wide QRS complex,
- The preceding RR interval usually is longer than the other ones
- Most aberrant beats are conducted via the left bundle branch, giving the appearance of right bundle branch block in lead V_1.
- The initial deflection of the wide QRS is in the same direction as that of the normal QRS complex.

An example of a supraventricular beat with aberrancy is shown in Figure 7-20

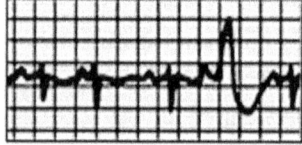

Figure 7-20. Supraventricular beat with aberrancy. Note the P wave preceding the wide QRS complex and the other indicators or aberration.

Ventricular Tachycardia

Ventricular tachycardia is defined as a run of three or more premature ventricular contractions. Figure 7-21 shows two sets of triplets.

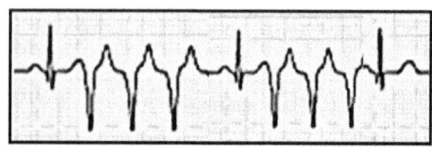

Figure 7-21. PVC triplets interspersed among normal heart beats.

The heart rate during ventricular tachycardia is usually 160 to 240 bpm.

Sustained ventricular tachycardia (Figure 7-22) is a life-threatening arrhythmia because patients are not able to maintain an adequate blood flow to vital organs.

The most common cause of V-tach is coronary artery disease, including myocardial infarction.

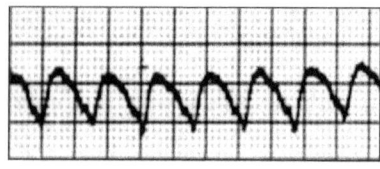

Figure 7-22. Ventricular tachycardia at a rate of about 225 bpm.

Supraventricular tachycardia in the presence of a bundle branch block may appear to be ventricular tachycardia. It may be difficult to tell the two apart. In an emergency, that which appears to be ventricular tachycardia is assumed to be so until proven otherwise.

Long QT Syndrome

Long QT syndrome (LQTS) is a disorder of the heart's electrical system. The condition leaves affected individuals vulnerable to the development of ventricular tachycardia which may lead, in some cases, to cardiac arrest and sudden death. The mechanism for the development of the ventricular tachycardia is felt to be the R on T phenomenon in which a premature ventricular complex lands on the T wave of the preceding beat; the longer the QT interval the greater the risk for developing ventricular tachycardia, such as Torsades de pointes (Figure 7-23). In French, Torsades de pointes means "Twisting of the points."

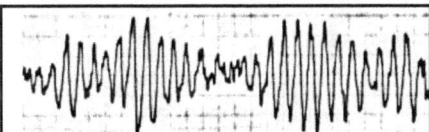

Figure 7-23. Torsades de pointes ventricular tachycardia.

Long QT syndrome can be genetic or caused by more than 50 medications, as well as electrolyte abnormalities and various medical conditions. Some of the causes of long QT syndrome are:

- Medications as mentioned in Chapter 1
- Congestive heart failure
- Electrolyte abnormalities (hypokalemia, hypocalcemia, hypomagnesemia)
- Hypothyroidism
- Myocardial ischemia and infarction
- Myocarditis
- Organophosphate insecticide poisoning
- Severe CNS events (CVA, seizures, intracranial hemorrhage)
- Slow heart rates
- Type Ia antiarrhythmic agents (quinidine, procainamide, disopyramide), as well as other antiarrhythmics
- Hereditary diseases (Jervell and Lang Nielson syndrome, Romano Ward syndrome)

Short QT Syndrome

The hallmark of *Short QT syndrome* is a QT interval of < 0.32 seconds that does not significantly change with heart rate. Tall, peaked T waves may be present. The heart is structurally normal. Some causes of short QT syndrome are:

- Medications (digoxin, rufinamide)
- Electrolyte abnormalities (hypercalcemia, hyperkalemia)
- Hypothermia
- Acidosis
- Sporadic occurrence
- Hereditary conditions

Individuals with short QT syndrome frequently complain of palpitations and may have syncope that is unexplained.

The hereditary form of short QT syndrome is inherited in an autosomal dominant pattern. Individuals typically have family members with a history of palpitations, atrial fibrillation, or sudden death at a young age, possibly including some cases of sudden infant death syndrome. Death is most likely due to ventricular fibrillation.

Ventricular Fibrillation

In *ventricular fibrillation (V-fib)* the ventricles do not beat in a coordinated fashion, but instead twitch asynchronously. Ventricular fibrillation is sometimes divided into coarse and fine rhythms. It is a potentially deadly arrhythmia because there is no cardiac output. An illustration of ventricular fibrillation is shown in Figure 7-24.

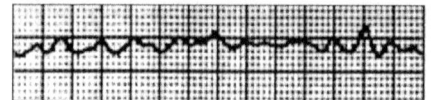

Figure 7-24. Ventricular fibrillation.

Asystole

Asystole is a cardiac arrest rhythm in which there is no discernible electrical activity on the ECG monitor (Figure 7-25). It often follows ventricular fibrillation.

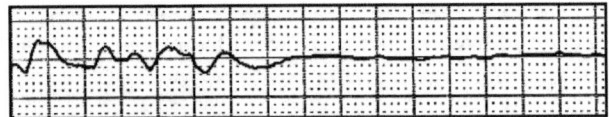

Figure 7-25. Asystole evolving from ventricular fibrillation.

Pulseless Electrical Activity

Pulseless electrical activity (PEA) is a clinical condition characterized by no palpable pulse but with some organized cardiac electrical activity. PEA was previously referred to as electromechanical dissociation. With both asystole and PEA there is no blood flow to the vital organs. Pulseless electrical activity can take many forms. One example is shown in figure 7-26.

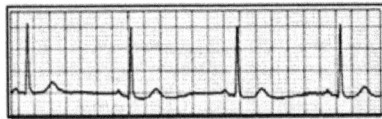

Figure 7-26. An example of pulseless electrical activity appearing as sinus bradycardia.

Idioventricular Rhythm

Since ventricular tissue is capable of spontaneous depolarization at an intrinsically slower rate than other areas of the heart, a ventricular focus may initiate depolarization when a faster pacemaker does not control the rate. Like junctional escape beats, ventricular escape beats occur after a pause in the regular rhythm. If a higher focus fails to pick up the rhythm, ventricular escape beats may continue. With a PVC a ventricular focus initiates depolarization when a faster pacemaker does not control the rate.

If a higher focus fails to pick up the rhythm, ventricular escape beats may continue. When this occurs, the rhythm is called *idioventricular rhythm* and has a rate usually 20 to 40 bpm. The QRS complex is wide and bizarre. P waves will, of course, not be present. An example of idioventricular rhythm is shown in Figure 7-27.

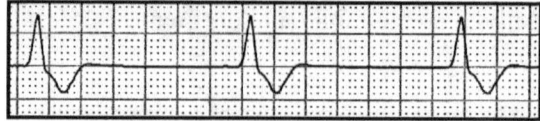

Figure 7-27. Idioventricular rhythm with a rate of about 40 bpm.

Idioventricular rhythms often are associated with increased vagal tone and decreased sympathetic tone. The rhythm classically is seen in the reperfusion phase of an acute STEMI; that is, post thrombolysis.

They usually are of short duration and as a rule require no intervention.

Accelerated idioventricular rhythms occur at a rate of 40 to 120 bpm (Figure 7-28). This distinguishes them from idioventricular rhythms with rates less than 40 and ventricular tachycardia with rates greater than 120.

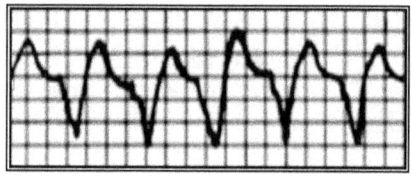

Figure 7-28. Accelerated idioventricular rhythm with a rate of about 80 bpm.

BIGEMINY

Bigeminy is an alternating pattern of combinations of atrial-atrial, atrial-ventricular, or ventricular-ventricular beats. Trigeminy and even *quadrigeminy* can occur. Figure 7-29A shows bigeminy consisting of atrial-atrial beats, Figure 7-29B shows bigeminy consisting of atrial-ventricular beats, and Figure 7-29C shows bigeminy with ventricular-ventricular beats

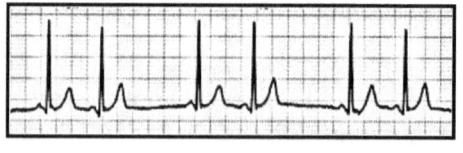

Figure 7-29A. Couplets of atrial beats.

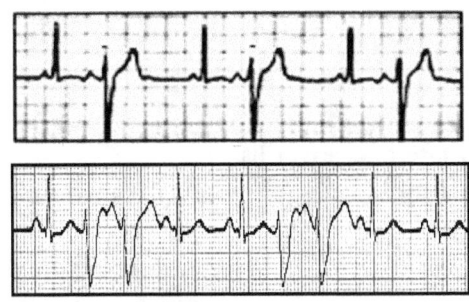

Figure 7-29B. Couplets of atrial and ventricular beats.

Figure 7-29C. Couplets of ventricular beats.

ELECTRICAL ALTERNANS

Electrical alternans (Figure 7-30) is technically not an arrhythmia, but occurs secondary to some underlying pathology. Most commonly it is associated with pericardial effusion, but also can occur secondary to pleural effusion or cardiac tamponade.

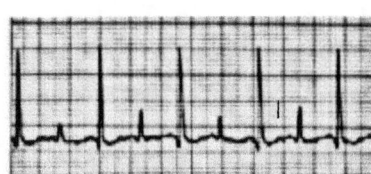

Figure 7-30. Electrical alternans due to pericardial tamponade

In the instance of pericardial effusion, the heart tends to move within the fluid with each contraction. When the motion of the heart within the effusion is increased, particularly when this is accompanied by tachycardia, the heart may not have returned to its previous position by the time the next cardiac cycle commences. Thus, with each depolarization the heart is in a slightly different position, and the QRS complex varies in intensity with each beat.

DIFFERENTIAL DIAGNOSIS OF TACHYCARDIA

Tachycardia can be divided into narrow complex tachycardia and wide complex tachycardia. These can be broken down further by whether the rhythm is regular or irregular (Table 7-1)

Table 7-1. Differential diagnosis of tachycardia.

	Narrow QRS complex	Wide QRS complex
Regular rhythm	Sinus tachycardia (ST) SVT Atrial flutter	ST with BBB SVT with BBB Ventricular tachycardia
Irregular rhythm	Atrial fibrillation (AF) with variable conduction Multifocal atrial tachycardia	AF with BBB AF with WPW Ventricular tachycardia

Chapter 7 Quiz

1. Name that rhythm!

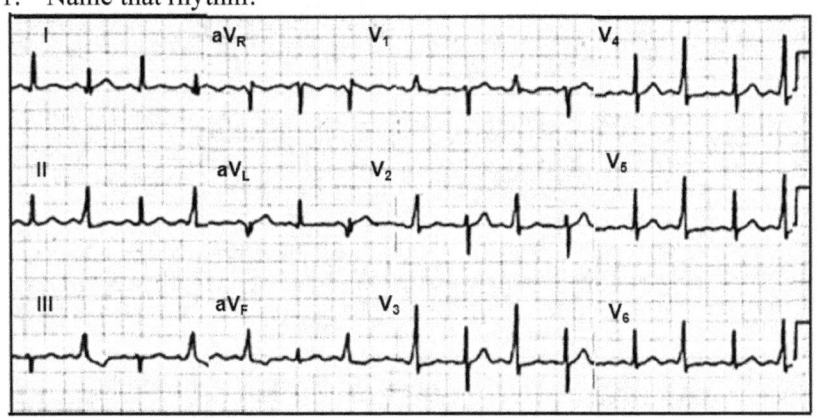

2. Name that rhythm!

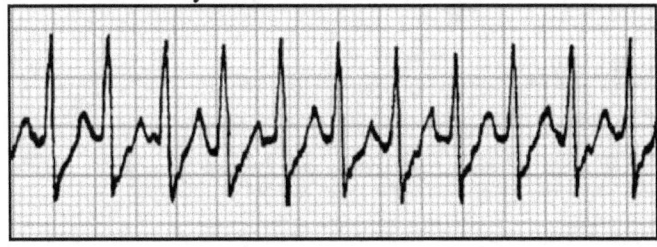

3. Name that rhythm!

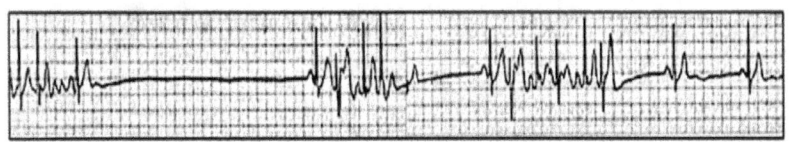

4. Name that rhythm!

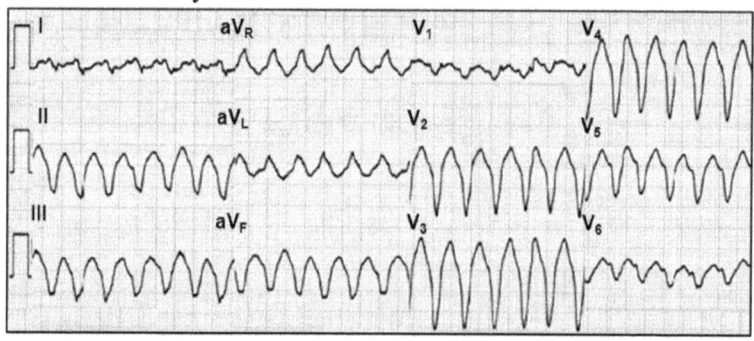

5. Name that rhythm!

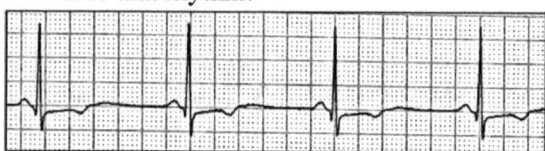

6. Name that rhythm!

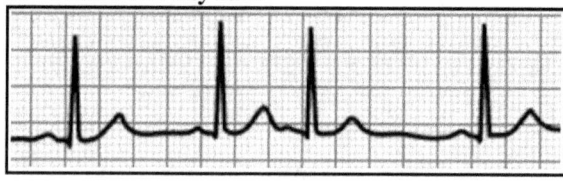

7. Name that rhythm!

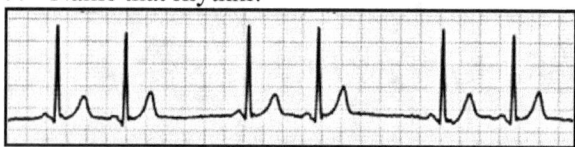

8. Name that rhythm!

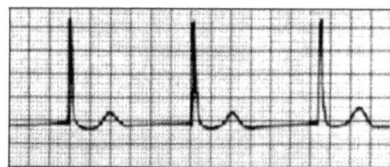

9. Name that rhythm!

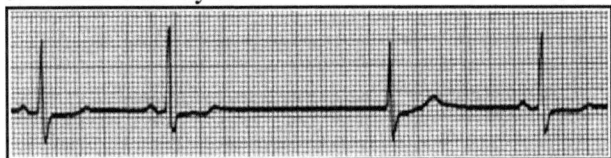

10. Name that rhythm!

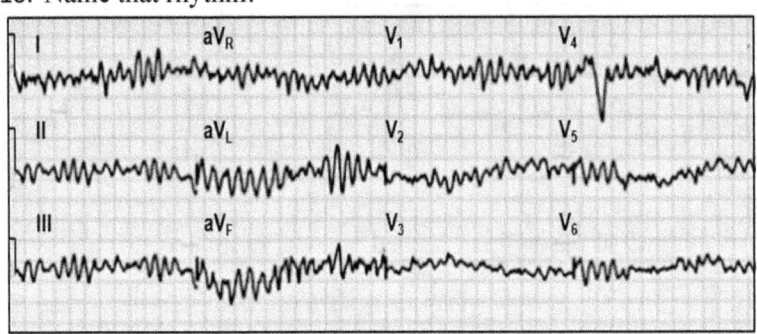

11. Name that rhythm!

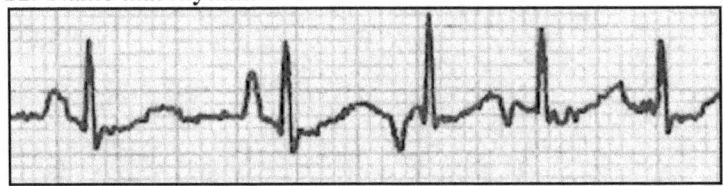

12. Name that rhythm!

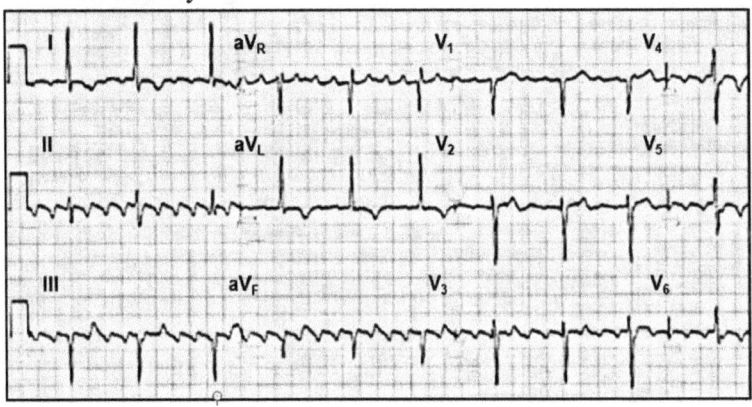

13. Name that rhythm!

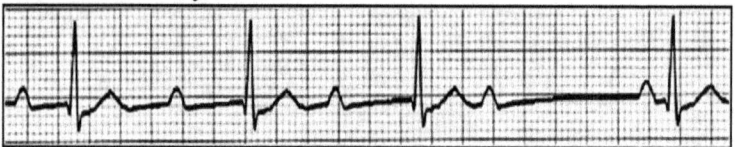

14. Name that rhythm!

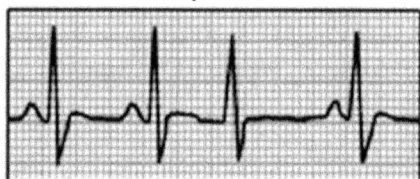

15. Name that rhythm!

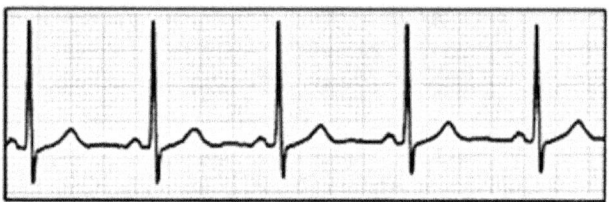

16. Name that rhythm!

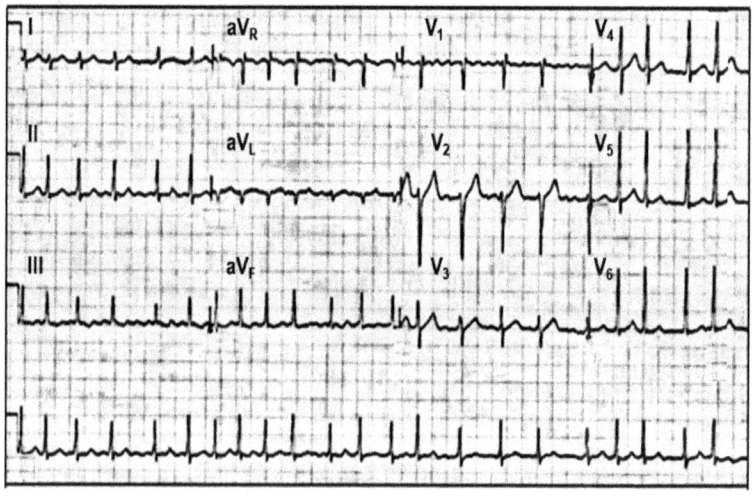

17. Name that rhythm!

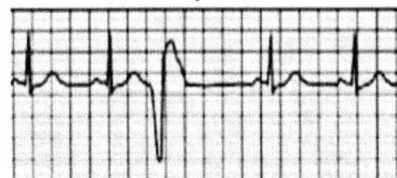

18. Name that rhythm!

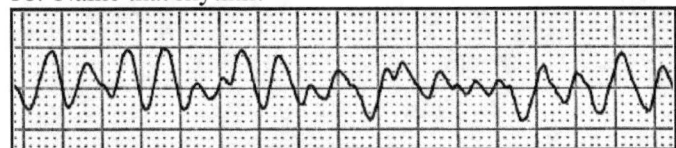

19. Name that rhythm!

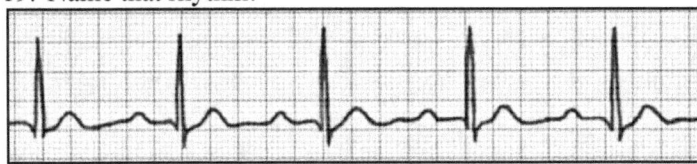

20. Name that rhythm!

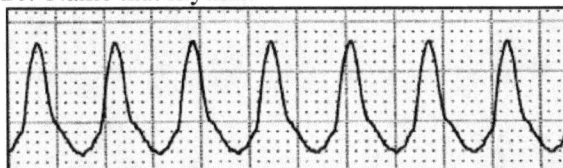

21. Name that rhythm!

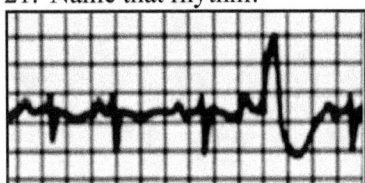

22. Name that rhythm!

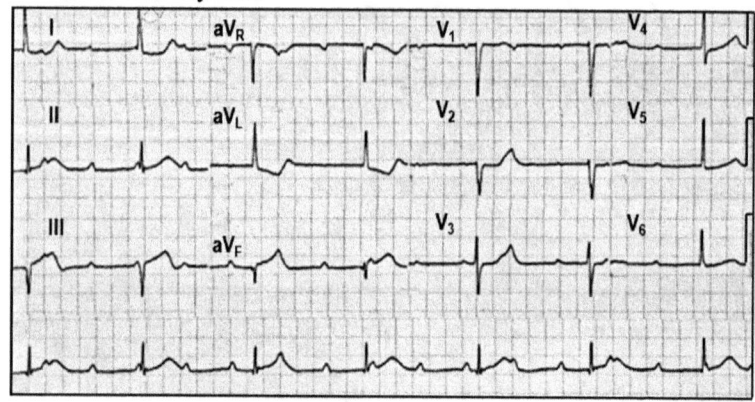

Chapter 8

Preexcitation Syndromes, Pulmonary Embolus, Pericarditis, Early Repolarization, and Myocarditis

As we saw in Chapter 1, the depolarization wave normally is initiated by the sinoatrial node. From there it passes down internodal fibers to the atrioventricular node, through the bundle of His, and down the right and left bundle branches. It should be remembered that this process normally requires 0.12 to 0.20 seconds, mostly because of slow passage in the atrioventricular node.

PREEXCITATION SYNDROMES

Preexcitation syndromes refer to clinical conditions in which the wave of depolarization initially bypasses the atrioventricular node as it passes from the atria to the ventricles. Because conduction through an accessory pathway is faster than that through the atrioventricular node, the time required for the wave to leave the sinoatrial node and arrive at ventricular muscle (PR interval) is shortened.

Two important preexcitation syndromes are Wolff-Parkinson-White syndrome and Lown-Ganong-Levine syndrome.

Wolff-Parkinson-White Syndrome

Patients with *Wolff-Parkinson-White (WPW) syndrome* possess an accessory pathway of depolarization known as the *bundle of Kent* (Figure 8-1). The bundle of Kent originates in atrial tissue and ends in ventricular muscle tissue. It may arise on the left or the right site of the heart. It is capable of rapidly conducting the depolarization wave from the atria, partially bypassing the delay in the atrioventricular node.

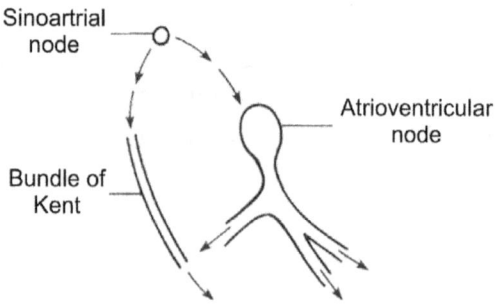

Figure 8-1. Accessory pathway of Wolff-Parkinson-White syndrome (bundle of Kent).

With Wolff-Parkinson-White syndrome, as atrial depolarization is being completed, the depolarization wave arrives simultaneously at the atrioventricular node and the atrial end of the bundle of Kent. Conduction through the atrioventricular node is delayed, but conduction passes rapidly through the bundle of Kent. After the initial focus of ventricular depolarization via the bundle of Kent has occurred, the remainder of the ventricular muscle is depolarized via the wave from the atrioventricular bundle. The net result is a QRS complex that is a composite of the initial premature ventricular depolarization and the later depolarization of the remaining myocardium via the normal conducting system. The early depolarization produces a slurring of the initial portion of the QRS complex called a *delta wave* as illustrated in Figure 8-2.

The three electrocardiographic criteria for Wolff-Parkinson-White syndrome are:

- Short PR interval (0.12 seconds or less)
- Wide QRS complex
- Delta wave (the QRS complex is widened by the delta wave exactly the same amount as the PR interval is shortened)

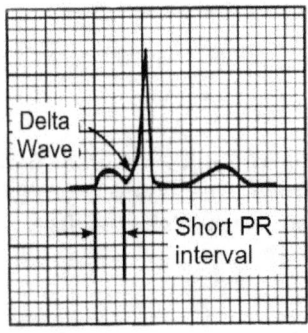

Figure 8-2. Electrocardiographic illustration of the Wolff-Parkinson-White syndrome.

The major clinical manifestation of Wolff-Parkinson-White syndrome is recurrent tachycardia due to the fact that the bundle of Kent allows the establishment of a continuous reentry cycle. The QRS complex may be normal or wide and bizarre depending on the direction of the reentry wave. If the atrioventricular node is depolarized in an antegrade fashion (orthodromic) and the bundle of Kent is activated retrograde, a normal QRS complex results (Figure 8-3A). However, if the atrioventricular node is depolarized in a retrograde fashion (antidromic) with antegrade depolarization of the bundle of Kent, a wide, bizarre QRS complex results (Figure 8-3B).

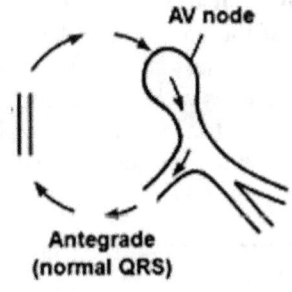

Figure 8-3A. Anterograde (orthodromic) reentry cycle of Wolff-Parkinson-White Syndrome.

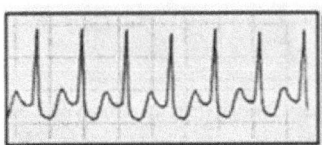

118

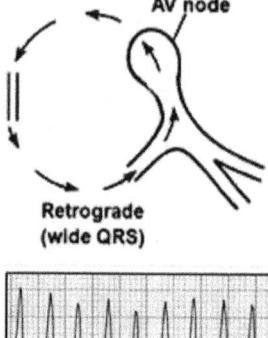

Figure 8-3B. Retrograde (anti-dromic) reentry cycle of Wolff-Parkinson-White Syndrome.

The accessory pathway of WPW syndrome can be on the right side of the heart or on the left side. WPW also can be classified as types A, B, and C.

- **Type A:** The delta waves are upright in all of the precordial leads.
- **Type B:** The delta waves are negative in leads V_1-V_3 and positive in leads V_4-V_6.
- **Type C:** The delta waves are positive in leads V_1-V_4 and negative in leads V_5-V_6

By the way, dromic means "like a racetrack."

Atrial fibrillation with Wolff-Parkinson-White Syndrome. The normal rate-limiting effects of the atrioventricular (AV) node are bypassed, and the resultant ventricular rates sometimes reaches 200 to 240 beats/minute. The ECG shows wide QRS complexes with a variable RR interval (Figure 8-4). Atrial fibrillation with Wolff-Parkinson-White Syndrome may lead to ventricular fibrillation and sudden death.

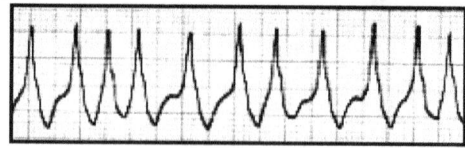

Figure 8.4. Atrial fibrillation with Wolff-Parkinson-White syndrome. Note the wide QRS complexes and the variable RR interval.

Lown-Ganong-Levine Syndrome

The *Lown-Ganong-Levine* syndrome is the result of some of the internodal fibers, called *James fibers*, bypassing the major portion of the atrioventricular node and terminating in the bundle of His as opposed to the ventricle muscle as in the WPW syndrome.

The major conduction delay in the atrioventricular node is partially bypassed by the James fibers (Figure 8-5).

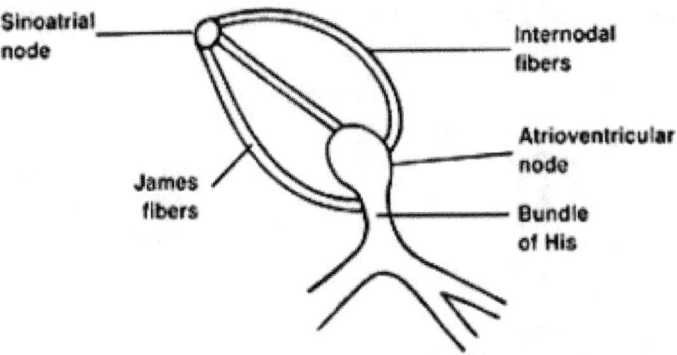

Figure 8-5. James fibers of Lown-Ganong-Levine syndrome terminating in the bundle of His.

The presence of the James fibers causes a short PR interval of less than 0.12 seconds. Ventricular depolarization takes place via the normal conduction pathway. Hence, the QRS complexes are of normal configuration (Figure 8-6).

The three criteria for Lown-Ganong-Levine syndrome are:

- A short PR interval less than 0.12 seconds without a delta wave
- A normal QRS complex
- A recurrent paroxysmal tachycardia

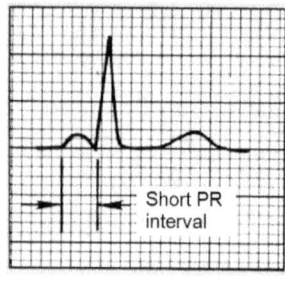

Figure 8-6. Electrocardiographic illustration of the Lown-Ganong-Levine syndrome.

The aberrant termination of internodal fibers can lead to a reentry depolarization wave (Figure 8-7), resulting in a supraventricular tachycardia with a normal-appearing QRS complex.

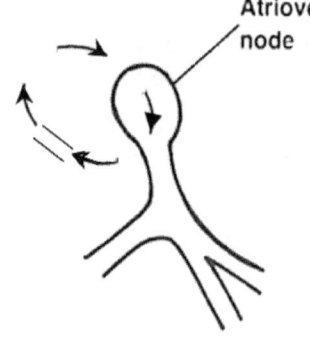

Figure 8-7. Reentry cycle of Lown-Ga-nong-Levine syndrome.

It should be noted that, unlike Wolff-Parkinson-White syndrome, episodes of tachycardia are required for the diagnosis of Lown-Ganong-Levine syndrome.

PULMONARY EMBOLUS

The ECG is abnormal with *pulmonary embolus* in more than two thirds of the cases, but findings are not sensitive or specific. The most common abnormal findings are sinus tachycardia and nonspecific ST segment and T wave changes. The $S_1Q_3T_3$ pattern (Figure 8-8) is a classic finding; however, it is present in only 10 percent of patients with a pulmonary embolus. The $S_1Q_3T_3$ pattern consists of:

- S wave in lead I
- Q wave in lead III
- T wave inversion in lead III

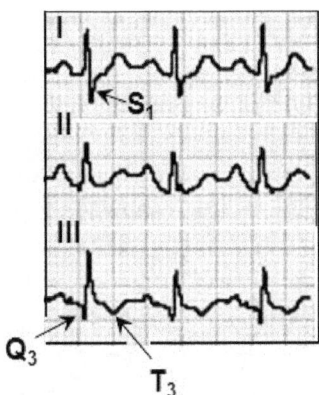

Figure 8.8. The $S_1Q_3T_3$ pattern of pulmonary embolus.

Other ECG findings of pulmonary embolus may include:

- Atrial fibrillation or other atrial arrhythmia
- Findings that mimic myocardial infarction (ST segment and T wave changes)
- Right axis deviation
- Right bundle branch block (transient)
- Right-sided strain pattern
- T wave inversion in precordial leads V_1-V_4

The bottom line is that the ECG is a poor diagnostic test for pulmonary embolism. The greatest utility of the procedure in the patient with suspected pulmonary embolism is ruling out other potential life-threatening diagnoses, such as myocardial infarction.

PERICARDITIS

Abnormal ECG findings are present in 90 percent of people with acute *pericarditis*. In general, changes may include:

- ST segment elevations (concave upward) and depressions

- PR segment depression, typically seen in lead II.
- ST/T ratios greater than 0.25 in the leads with ST segment elevations, a finding frequently indicative of acute pericarditis
- Reciprocal ST segment depressions for the ST segment elevations are not seen.
- ST segment elevation may be present in all leads
- Sinus tachycardia is common and is due to pain and/or pericardial effusion.

Pericarditis usually follows a recent viral illness. An ECG from a patient with acute viral pericarditis is shown in Figure 8-9.

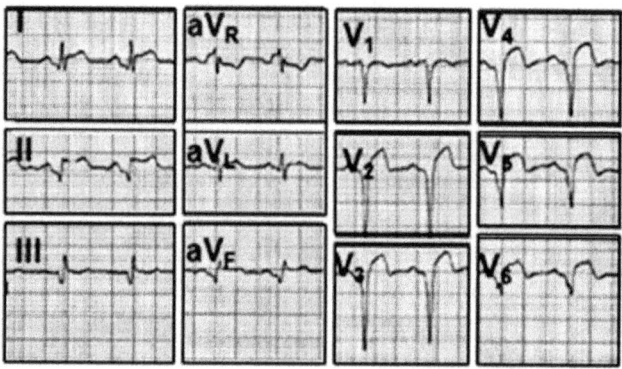

Figure 8-9. Acute pericarditis. Note the PR segment depressions in leads I and II, the ST segment elevations in leads V₂-V₆, and the ST/T ratio greater than 0.25.

Stages of Pericarditis

The ECG in acute viral pericarditis typically shows changes that evolve through four stages over a period of three to four weeks. About 50 percent of patients with pericarditis demonstrate all four phases.

Stage I. *Stage I pericarditis* (Figure 8-10A) is characterized by an onset of one to two days and a duration of up to two weeks. Electrocardiograph changes are as above.

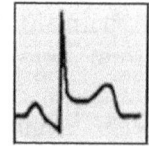

Stage II. *Stage II pericarditis* (Figure 8-10B) is characterized by a duration of days to weeks. During this period of time the ST segments return toward baseline and the T waves flatten.

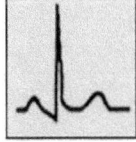

Stage III. *Stage III pericarditis* (Figure 8-10C) begins by week two or three and has a duration of two to three weeks. Electrocardiographic findings include a return of ST segments to baseline and deep T wave inversions in leads II, aV_F, and V_4-V_6.

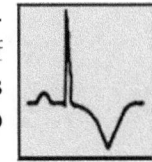

Stage IV. *Stage IV pericarditis* (Figure 8-10D) is characterized by a duration of up to three months, with gradual resolution of T wave inversions and return of the ECG to normal.

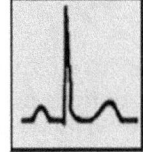

EARLY REPOLARIZATION

Early repolarization is a common finding in young, healthy individuals. It tends to disappear with advancing age. It is more prominent in the precordial leads (Figure 8-11). It appears as mild ST segment elevations that can be diffuse.

Characteristics of early repolarization include:

- Concave ST segment elevations (< 3 mm) in leads V_2-V_5.
- The ST segment elevation in this setting appears as an elevated J point.
- The ST elevations tend to decrease in magnitude with increasing heart rate due to sympathetic stimulation.
- There are no reciprocal ST segment depressions to suggest STEMI.
- Large symmetrically concordant T waves are present in leads with ST segment elevation.
- T waves may be peaked.
- Terminal QRS notching or slurring may occur.
- No PR segment depressions as in pericarditis.

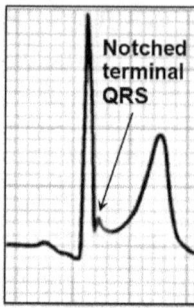

Figure 8-11. Early repolarization. Note the notched terminal QRS, elevated J point, and ST segment elevation with a concave shape.

Three things may help distinguish early repolarization from pericarditis:

1. *ST/T ratio* less than 0.25 in the leads with ST segment elevations (early repolarization).
2. The ST elevation in early repolarization resolves when the person exercises.
3. Early repolarization, unlike pericarditis, is a benign ECG finding that should not be associated with symptoms.

Table 8-1 compares the ECG findings of pericarditis to those of STEMI and early repolarization.

Table 8.1. Comparison of acute pericarditis to STEMI and early repolarization.

ECG Finding	Acute Pericarditis	STEMI	Early Repolarization
ST segment shape	Concave upward	Convex upward	Concave upward
Q waves	Absent	Present	Absent
Reciprocal ST segment changes	Absent	Present	Absent
Location of ST segment elevation	Limb and chest leads	Area of involved myocardium	Chest leads
PR segment depression	Present	Absent	Absent

MYOCARDITIS

Myocarditis is an inflammatory disease of the heart muscle that can result from a variety of causes. While most cases are produced by a viral infection, inflammation of the heart muscle may also be caused by toxins, drugs, and immune reactions.

ECG findings most commonly seen with myocarditis are:

- Diffuse T wave inversions
- ST segment elevations without reciprocal depressions.
- Low voltage QRS complexes.
- Atrial and ventricular ectopic beats, atrial and ventricular tachycardia, or atrial fibrillation may be present.
- Heart block may be observed.

An ECG from a patient with myocarditis is shown in Figure 8-12.

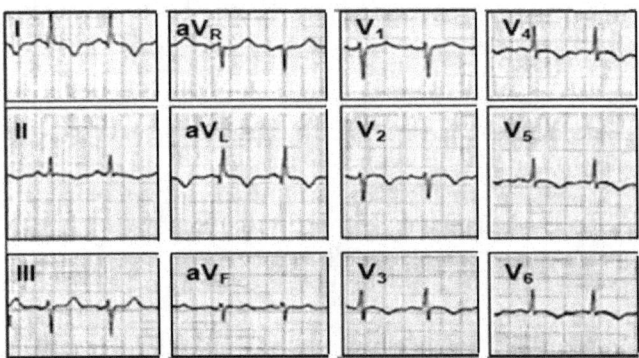

Figure 8-12. ECG of a patient with myocarditis. Note the diffuse T wave inversions and low-voltage QRS complexes.

The ECG changes of myocarditis may persist for several months before they resolve spontaneously.

Chapter 8 Quiz

1. A tachyarrhythmia is required for the diagnosis of WPW syndrome (T or F).

2. Orthodromic nodal conduction is clockwise or counter clockwise?

3. What is your diagnosis?

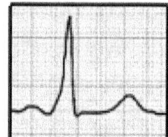 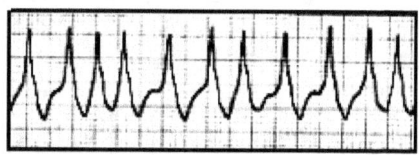

4. A tachyarrhythmia is required for the diagnosis of LGL syndrome (T or F).

5. 5. The $S_1Q_3T_3$ pattern with pulmonary embolus is present _____ percent of the time.
   A. 10
   B. 20
   C. 30
   D. 40

6. The ST segment elevation with early repolarization appears as an elevated J point in which:
   A. ST/T > 0.25
   B. ST/T < 0.25
   C. ST/T = 0.25
   D. None of the above

Interpret the following ECGs. Use the 8 steps discussed in Chapter 1.

7. History of tachycardia

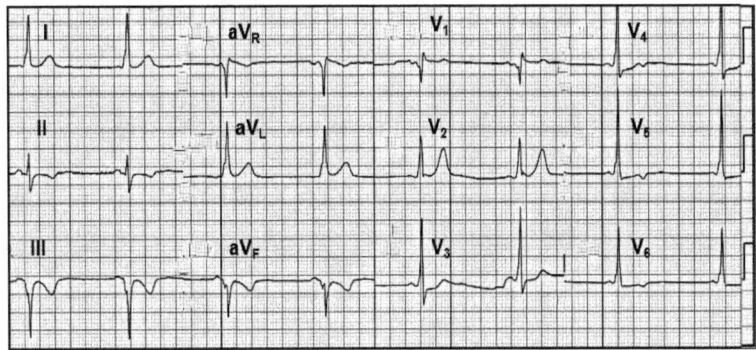

8.

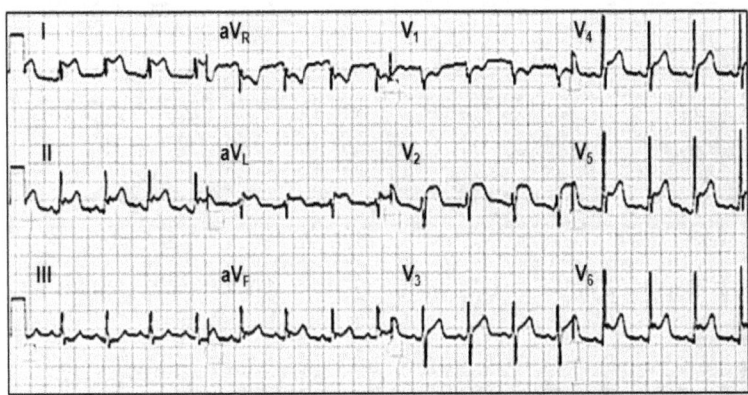

9.

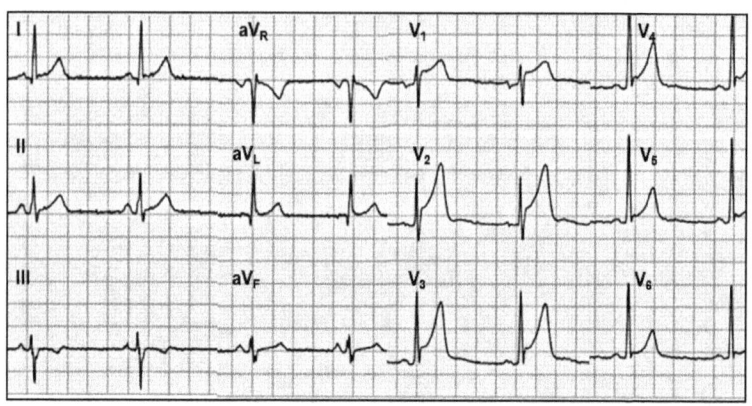

10. Patient has had spells of tachycardia

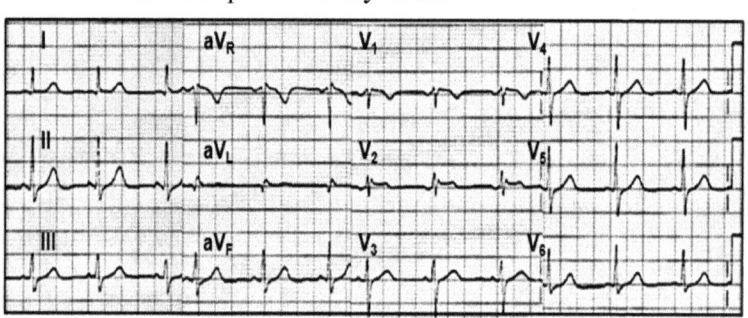

11. Patient has chest pain and fever

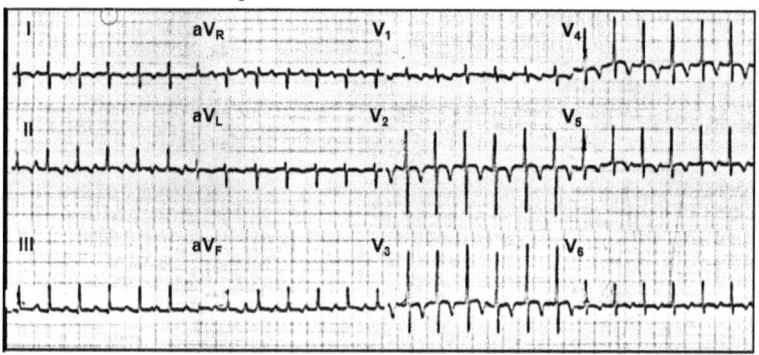

12.

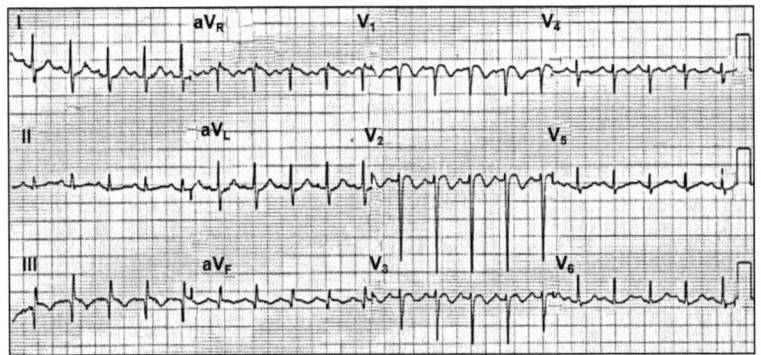

Chapter 9

Hypothermia, Low Voltage ECG, Neurological Insult, Dextrocardia, Pacemakers, Takotsumo Cardiomyopathy, Brugada Syndrome, and Arrhythmogenic Right Ventricular Dysplasia

HYPOTHERMIA

Hypothermia is a potentially fatal condition. It occurs when body temperature falls below 35° C (95° F). Figure 9-1 shows an ECG of a person with hypothermia.

The ECG findings of hypothermia include:

- Low voltage.
- Bradycardia with lengthening of all segments
- A baseline artifact from shivering may be present
- Osborn waves may be present

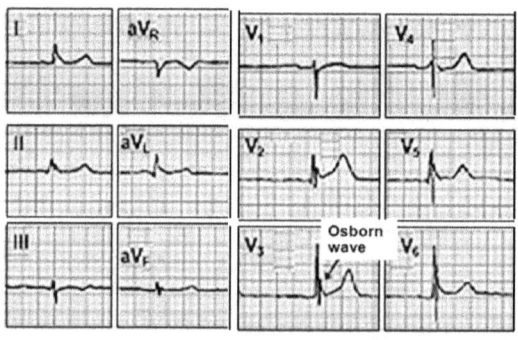

Figure 9-1. Hypothermia. Note the low voltage, bradycardia, and Osborn waves. A shivering artifact is not present.

An Osborn wave is characterized by a notch in the downward portion of the R wave in the QRS complex. It is in the same direction as the QRS complex and roughly proportional to the degree of hypothermia.

LOW VOLTAGE ECG

Low voltage on the ECG is defined as a peak-to-peak QRS amplitude of < 5 mm in the limb leads and/or < 10 mm in the precordial leads. Low voltage ECG may be present in the following situations:

- Half standard (when full standard is incorrectly expected)
- Obesity (fat tissue between the heart and the chest wall)
- Pericardial effusion
- Severe hypothyroidism
- Subcutaneous emphysema
- Massive myocardial damage/infarction
- Infiltrative/restrictive diseases such as amyloid
- Pulmonary emphysema
- Pleural effusion
- Pneumothorax

Figure 9-2 Shows a low voltage ECG from a patient with emphysema.

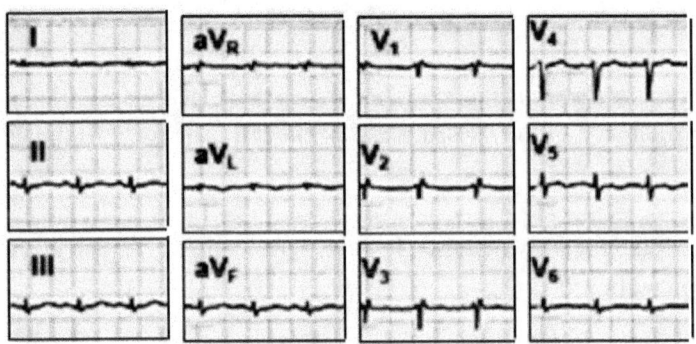

Figure 9-2. Low voltage ECG from a patient with emphysema.

NEUROLOGICAL INSULT

Most commonly seen in the setting of acute stroke, intracranial hemorrhage, or subarachnoid hemorrhage, neurologic injury can result in the following ECG changes:

- Diffuse, deeply inverted T waves
- Prolonged QT interval
- Bradyarrhythmias

These changes may mimic ischemia. The changes are shown in Figure 9-3.

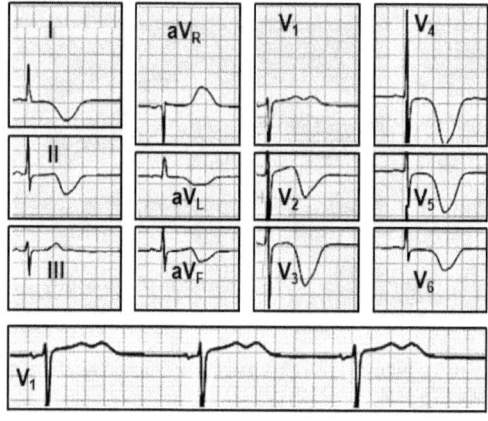

Figure 9-3. ECG of patient who suffered a cerebral hemorrhage. Note the deeply inverted T waves and prolonged QT interval. The rhythm strip at the bottom shows a sinus bradycardia of about 30 bpm.

DEXTROCARDIA

Dextrocardia (situs inversus) occurs when the heart is positioned in the right side of the chest instead of the left. The ECG findings include:

- Predominantly negative P wave, QRS complex, and T wave in lead I
- Low voltages in leads V_3-V_6

Figure 9-4 shows the ECG of a person with dextrocardia.

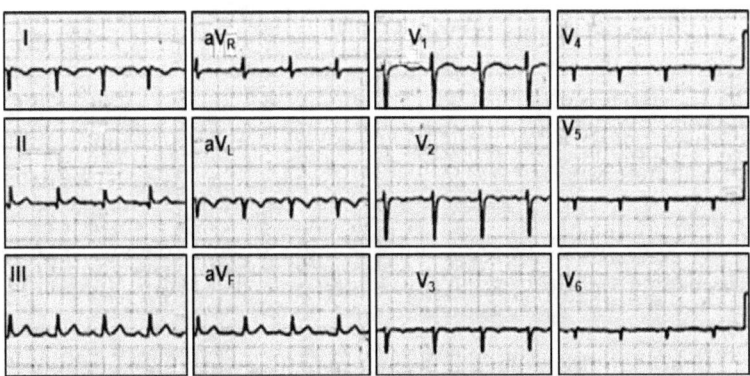

Figure 9-4. Dextrocardia showing negative P wave, QRS complex, and T wave in lead I and low voltages in leads V3-V6.

PACEMAKERS

Pacemakers are battery-powered, implantable devices that electrically stimulate the heart, causing the ventricles to contract and pump blood throughout the body. A pacemaker consists of a device which contains a battery and the electronic circuitry that runs the pacemaker and one or more long thin wires that travel through a vein in the chest to the heart. Pacemakers are usually implanted in patients in whom the heart's sinoatrial node is no longer functioning normally.

The appearance of the ECG in a paced patient is dependent on pacing mode, placement of pacing leads, device pacing thresholds, and the presence of native electrical activity.

With atrial pacing, the pacemaker spike precedes the P wave. The shape of the P wave depends on the placement of the lead, but may appear normal (Figure 9-5).

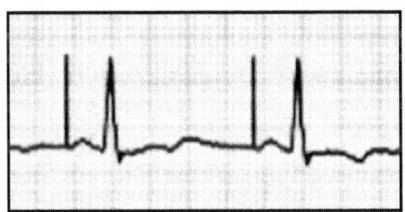

Figure 9-5. Atrial pacemaker. Note the pacemaker spike before the P wave.

With ventricular pacing, the pacing spike precedes the QRS complex. Right ventricle pacing results in a QRS morphology similar to LBBB. Left ventricular pacing results in a QRS morphology similar to RBBB. ST segments and T waves are discordant with the QRS complex.

With dual chamber pacing the ECG appearance depends on the areas being paced. It may exhibit features of atrial pacing, ventricular pacing, or both. Pacing spikes may precede P waves, QRS complexes, or both.

Figure 9-6 shows the ECG evidence of a ventricular pacemaker. Note the spikes created by the pacemaker firings, the wide QRS complexes, and the discordance of the QRS complexes and the T waves.

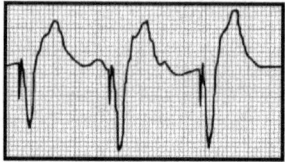

Figure 9-6. Ventricular pacemaker. Note the pacemaker spike before the QRS complex.

With dual chamber pacing the ECG appearance depends on the areas being paced. It may exhibit features of atrial pacing, ventricular pacing, or both (Figure 9-7). Pacing spikes may precede P waves, QRS complexes, or both.

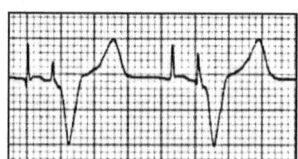

Figure 9-7. Atrial/ventricular pacemaker. Note the pacemaker spikes before the P waves and QRS complexes.

TAKOTSUBO CARDIOMYOPATHY

Takotsubo cardiomyopathy (stress induced cardiomyopathy, broken heart syndrome, apical ballooning syndrome) is a rare condition that consists of transient systolic dysfunction of the left apical and/or left midventricular segments of the heart. It has an abrupt onset and is usually triggered by a stressful event, such as the death of a loved one or a romantic break up. It usually occurs in middle-aged or older women. A sudden high level of circulating catecholamines is felt to be responsible.

The condition is characterized by chest pain, shortness of breath, and ECG changes that mimic myocardial infarction. Coronary artery disease is not present. ECG changes may include:

- ST segment elevation
- ST segment depression
- Prolonged QT interval

Figure 9-8 shows the ECG of a patient with Takotsubo cardiomyopathy.

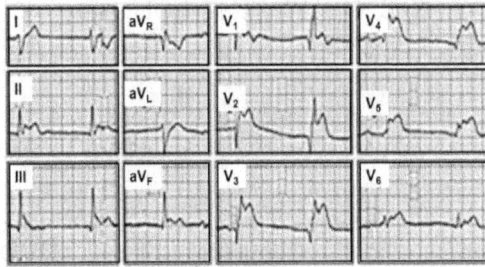

Figure 9-8. ECG of a patient with Takotsubo cardiomyopathy. Note the ST segment elevations and depressions.

BRUGADA SYNDROME

Brugada syndrome is a genetic disorder that results in sudden cardiac death from polymorphic ventricular tachycardia or ventricular fibrillation in the setting of a structurally normal heart. Unlike other genetic syndromes that result in sudden cardiac death the QT interval in Brugada syndrome is normal.

There are three types of Brugada syndrome. The ECG findings of the three are as follow:

- **Type I:** Lead V_1 has a coved ST segment elevation of at least 2 mm followed by a negative T wave
- **Type II:** There is a saddleback appearance of the ST segment in lead V_1 with ST elevation of at least 2 mm. This can be present in normal individuals as well.
- **Type III:** Features of type I (coved) or type II (saddleback) with < 2 mm of ST segment elevation.

Brugada syndrome types are shown in Figure 9-9. Treatment of Brugada syndrome is an implantable cardioverter defibrillator (ICD).

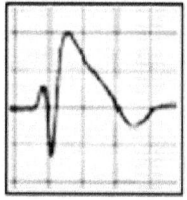 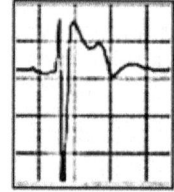 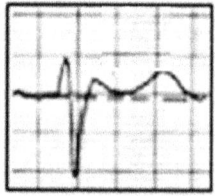

Coved ST segment Saddleback ST segment Coved and saddleback ST segment

Figure 9-9. Brugada syndrome Types.

ARRHYTHMOGENIC RIGHT VENTRICULAR DYSPLASIA

Arrhythmogenic right ventricular dysplasia (ARVD) occurs when the muscle tissue in the right ventricle dies and is replaced with scar tissue. This disrupts the heart's electrical signal and causes arrhythmias. Symptoms include palpitations and fainting after physical activity. It can cause sudden cardiac arrest in young athletes. ARVD usually affects teens or young adults and is thought to be congenital. ECG findings of ARVD may include:

- Epsilon wave (Figure 9-10)
- T wave inversions in V_1-V_3
- Prolonged S-wave upstroke in V_1-V_3
- Localized QRS widening in V_1-V_3
- Paroxysmal episodes of ventricular tachycardia with LBBB morphology

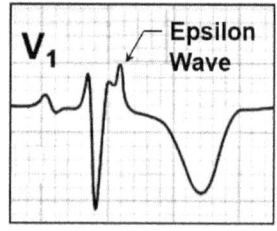

Figure 9-10. Epsilon wave of arrhythmogenic right ventricular dysplasia (seen in 50 percent of patients). Note the T wave inversion.

Chapter 9 Quiz

1. Hypothermia results in a baseline shivering artifact:
   A. Always
   B. Sometimes
   C. Never
   D. Every other case of hypothermia

2. Neurologic injury results in:
   A. Diffuse, markedly peaked T waves
   B. Shortened QT intervals
   C. Tachyarrhythmias
   D. Bradyarrhythmias

3. Dextrocardia (situs inversus) ECG findings include low voltage in leads:
   A. I, II, and III
   B. II, III, and aVF
   C. V_4, V_5, and V_6
   D. aV_R, aV_L, and aV_F

4. Takotsubo cardiomyopathy always occurs with the presence of underlying coronary artery disease (T or F)

5. The QT interval is normal or prolonged in Brugada syndrome.

Interpret the following ECGs. Use the 8 steps discussed in Chapter 1.

6.

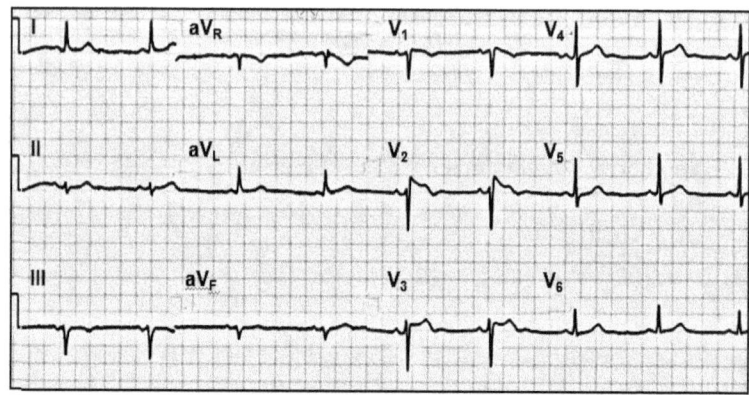

7.

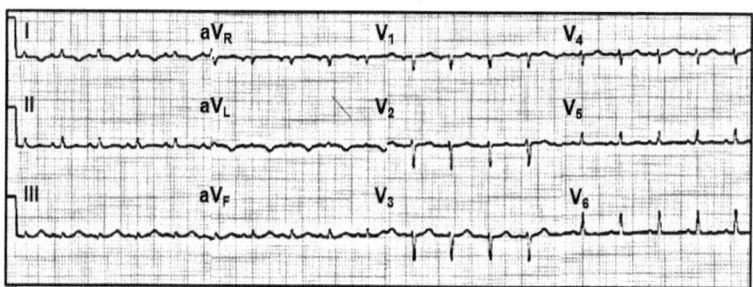

8.

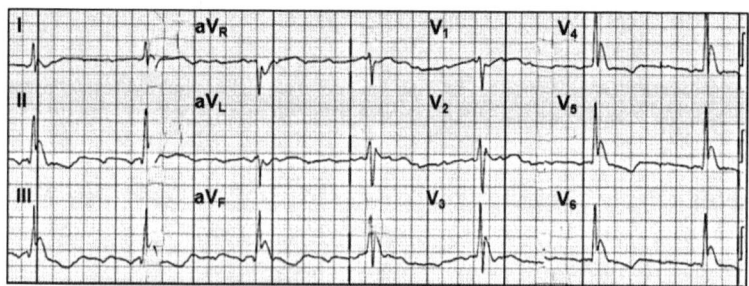

9.

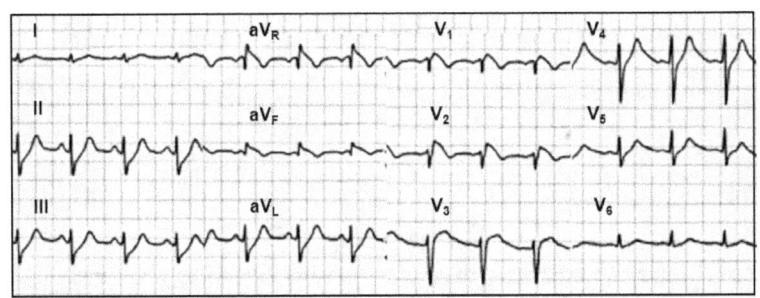

10.

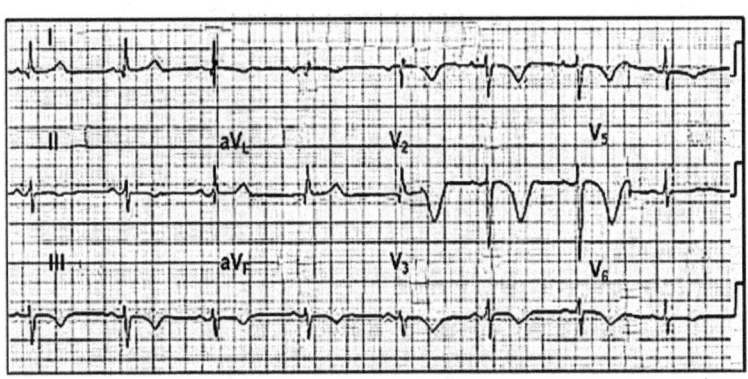

11.

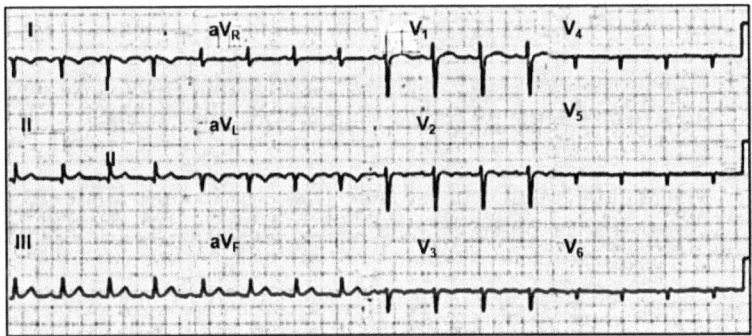

Chapter 10

Drug Effects, Electrolyte Effects, and ECG Worksheet

MEDICATION EFFECTS

Digoxin

Digoxin Effect

Digoxin effect occurs in the therapeutic range and may include:

- Increased automaticity (arrhythmias)
- AV block (long PR interval)
- Short QT
- Scooped ST-T complex
- The ST segment and T wave are fused together and it is impossible to tell where one ends and the other begins.

Digoxin effect is shown in Figure 10-1. The scooped ST segment is often said to resemble the mustache of Salvadore Dali, a Spanish artist (1904–1989).

Digoxin effect should be distinguished from digoxin toxicity.

Digoxin Toxicity

Changes in the electrocardiogram due to toxic levels of digoxin include:

- Virtually any arrhythmia (PVCs, regular or slow atrial fibrillation, ventricular tachycardia).
- All degrees of atrioventricular block

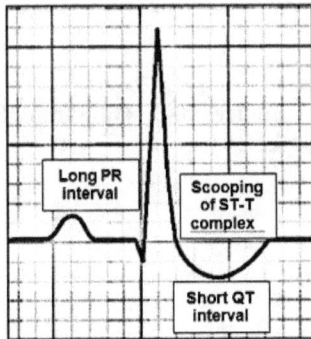

Figure 10-1. Effects of digoxin.

Bidirectional ventricular tachycardia is a rare dysrhythmia characterized by a beat-to-beat alternation of the QRS axis (Figure 10-2). It is most commonly seen with digoxin toxicity.

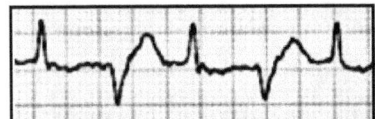

Figure 10-2. Bidirectional ventricular tachycardia.

Quinidine

Quinidine Effect

The effect of therapeutic doses of class 1a (quinidine, procainamide, disopyramide) and class 1c (flecainide, propafenone) antiarrhythmic agents decreases the automaticity of the SA node. Their effects on the ECG are classically known as the quinidine effect and may include:

- Decrease in the amplitude of the T waves or T wave inversions
- ST segment depression
- Prominent U waves
- Prolongation of the QT interval

- Notching and widening of the P waves

Some quinidine effects are shown in Figure 10-3.

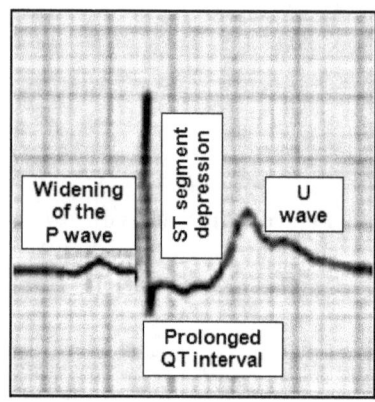

Figure 10-3. Quinidine Effect.

Quinidine Toxicity

Changes in the electrocardiogram due to toxic levels of type 1a antiarrhythmics may include:

- Widening of the QRS complex
- Various degrees of AV block
- Ventricular arrhythmias, syncope, and sudden death
- Marked sinus bradycardia, sinus arrest, or SA block

Some effects of quinidine toxicity are shown in Figure 10-4.

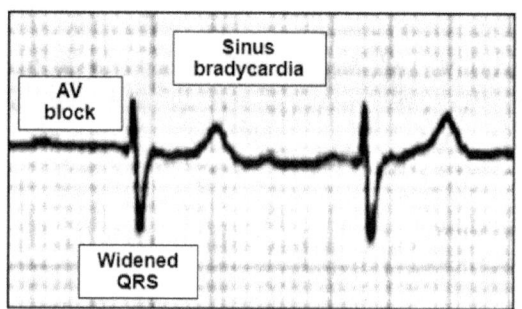

Figure 10-4. Quinidine toxicity.

Tricyclic Antidepressants

Tricyclic antidepressant overdose is characterized by:

* Sinus Tachycardia
* Terminal R wave $\geq$ 3 mm in aV_R
* Wide QRS
* Long QT

These changes are shown in Figure 10-5.

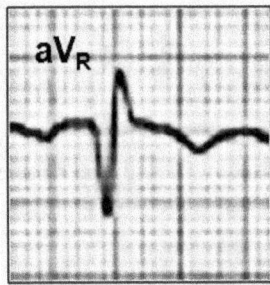

Figure 10-5. ECG changes of tricyclic overdose in lead aV_R.

Beta Blocker and Calcium Channel Blocker Toxicity

Beta blockers and calcium channel blockers in excess can have the following effects on the ECG:

* Sinus bradycardia.
* 1st degree, 2nd degree, and 3rd degree AV block.
* Junctional bradycardia.
* Ventricular bradycardia.

Hypomagnesemia

The primary ECG abnormality that may be seen with hypomagnesemia is prolonged QTc. Atrial and ventricular ectopy, atrial tachyarrhythmias, and torsades de pointes also may be seen but whether or not these effects are the result of concurrent hypokalemia is uncertain.

ELECTROLYTE EFFECTS

Potassium

Hyperkalemia produces:

- Tall, peaked T waves
- Widening of the QRS complex
- Prolongation of the PR interval

In higher levels, hyperkalemia produces:

- Loss of P waves
- Spread of the QRS complex into a smooth, continuous sine wave.

There is a rough correlation between the degree of change in the electrocardiogram and the concentration of potassium in the serum, as can be seen in Figure 10-6.

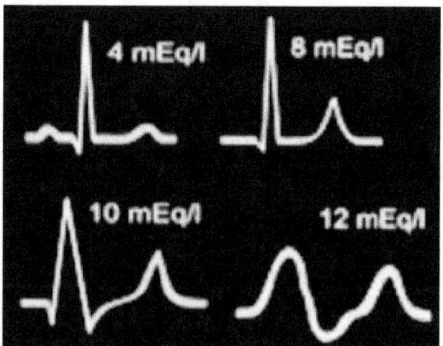

Figure 10-6. Correlations between serum potassium levels and the electrocardiogram in hyperkalemia.

Hypokalemia produces:

- Flattening of the T waves, which may unmask U waves
- T waves may become inverted
- ST segment depression may occur

- Increased amplitude and flattening of P wave
- Prolongation of PR interval

Some effects of hypokalemia on the ECG are shown in Figure 10-7.

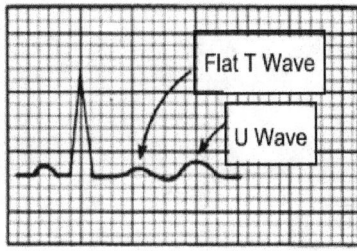

Figure 10-7. Some effects of hypokalemia on the electro-cardiogram.

Calcium

Hypercalcemia shortens ventricular repolarization time, resulting in a shortened QT interval (Figure 10-8A). *Hypocalcemia* prolongs the QT interval (Figure 10-8B).

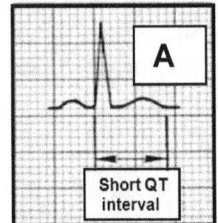
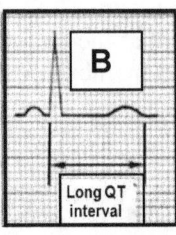

Figure 10-8. Effects of (A) hypercalcemia and (B) hypocalcemia on the electro-cardiogram.

ECG WORKSHEET

Electrocardiograms must be read in an orderly fashion. It is helpful to use a worksheet, such as the one presented in Table 10-1. One observes (1) the calibration to determine if the ECG is full or half standard, (2) rate, (3) rhythm, (4) axis, (5) intervals/segments, (6) signs of ventricular hypertrophy or atrial enlargement, (7) signs of infarction or ischemia, and (8) any other observations.

Table 10-1. A worksheet for collating electrocardiographic findings to facilitate interpretation.

1. Standard: Half _____ Full_____
2. Rate: Atrial _____ bpm   Ventricular _____ bpm
3. Rhythm:
   Regular: Yes _____   No _____
   Irregularly regular: Yes _____   No _____
   Irregularly irregular: Yes _____   No _____
4. Axis:
   Normal range _____   RAD zone _____   LAD zone _____
   Northwest axis zone _____
5. Intervals:
   PR _____ seconds
   QRS _____ seconds
   QT _____ seconds   QTc _____ seconds
   PR segment depression: Yes _____   No _____
6. Atrial enlargement: RAE _____ LAE _____ BAE _____
   Ventricular hypertrophy: RVH _____ LVH _____ BVH _____
7. ST segment elevations: Leads _____
   ST segment depressions: Leads _____
   Q waves: Leads: _____
   R wave progression: Normal _____ Abnormal _____
8. Other _____
   Interpretation _____

PRACTICE ECG

Practice reading the ECG in Figure 10-9. Record your responses in Table 10-1. The history is that the patient, a 56-year-old white male who presented to the emergency room of his local hospital 45 minutes after the onset of severe chest pain and nausea but no vomiting.

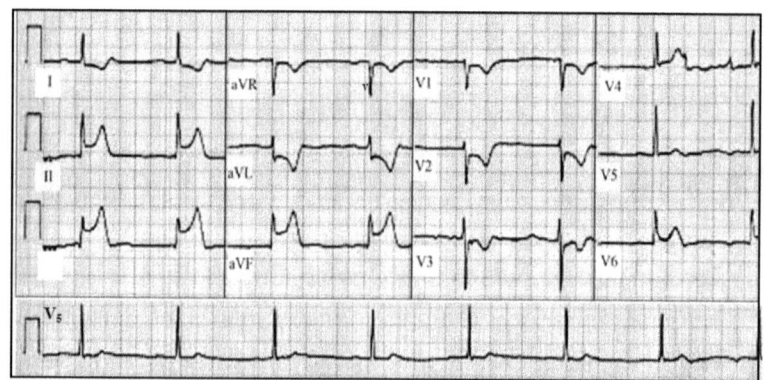

Figure 10-9. Practice ECG. Record your results in Table 10-1.

The results for the electrocardiogram of Figure 10-9 are given in Table 10-2.

Table 10-2. Results for ECG in Figure 10-7

1. Standard: Half _____ Full __x__
2. Rate: Atrial ___50___ bpm   Ventricular ___50___ bpm
3. Rhythm:
   Regular: Yes __x__ No _____
   Irregularly regular: Yes _____ No _____
   Irregularly irregular: Yes _____ No _____
4. Axis:
   Normal range __X__ RAD zone _____ LAD zone _____
   Northwest axis zone _____
5. Intervals:
   PR ___0.28___ seconds
   QRS ___0.08___ seconds
   QT ___0.40___ seconds QTc __0.38__ seconds
   PR segment depression: Yes _____ No __x__
6. Atrial enlargement: RAE __no__ LAE __no__ BAE __no__
   Ventricular hypertrophy: RVH __no__ LVH __no__ BVH __no__
7. ST segment elevations: Leads _____II, III, aV$_F$_____
   ST segment depressions: Leads _____I, aV$_L$, V$_1$-V$_2$_____
   Q waves: Leads: _____none_____
   R wave progression: Normal __x__ Abnormal _____
8. Other _____
Interpretation _____inferior STEMI_____

Chapter 10 Quiz

1. *Digoxin effect* occurs in the therapeutic range and may include all but:
   A. Increased automaticity (arrhythmias)
   B. AV block (long PR interval)
   C. Long QT interval
   D. Scooped ST-T complex

2. The *quinidine effect* may include all but:
   A. Notching and widening of the P waves
   B. Decrease in the amplitude of the T wave or T wave inversion
   C. ST segment elevation
   D. Prominent U waves
   E. Prolongation of the QT interval

3. Tricyclic overdose can result in all but:
   A. Sinus bradycardia
   B. Terminal R wave $\geq$ 3 mm in aV_R
   C. Long QT
   D. R/S ratio > 0.7 in aVR
   E. Wide QRS

4. Hyperkalemia at 10 mEq results in all but:
   A. Prolonged PR interval
   B. Prolonged QRS
   C. Prolonged QT interval
   D. Tall T waves

5. Hypercalcemia results in a long or short QT interval.

Interpret the following ECGs

6.

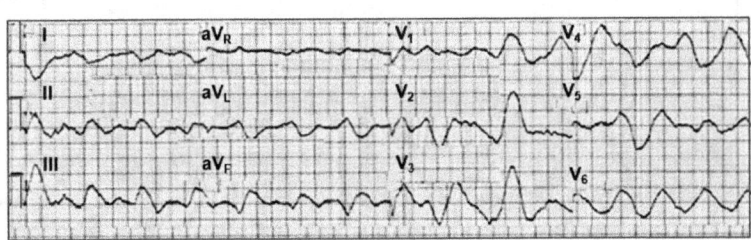

7.

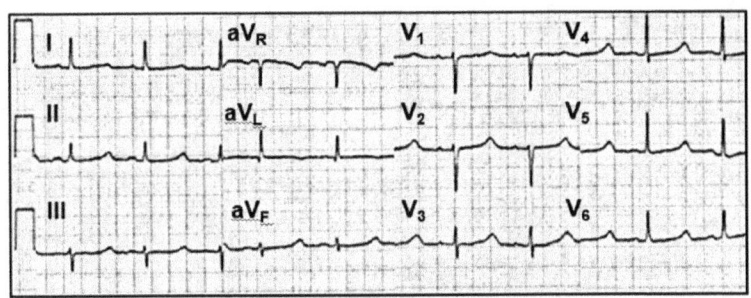

8.

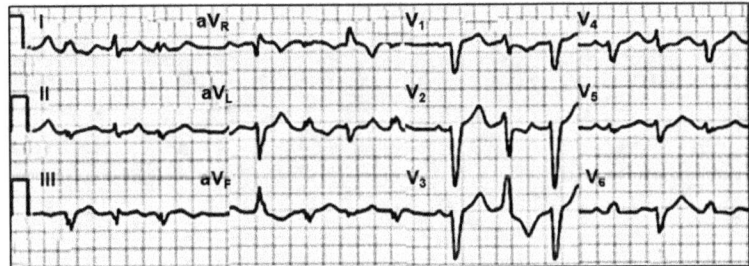

9.

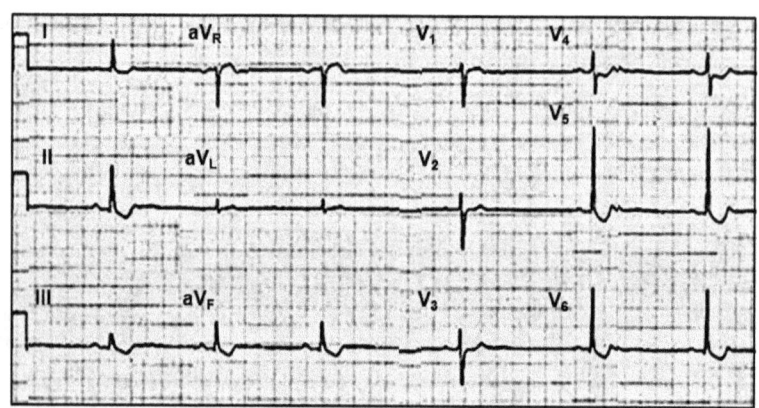

10.

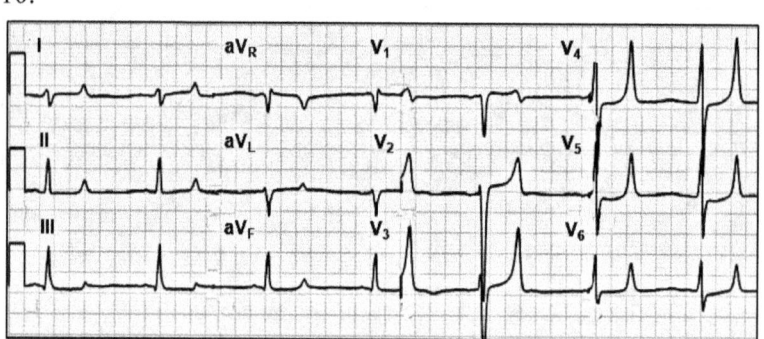

11.

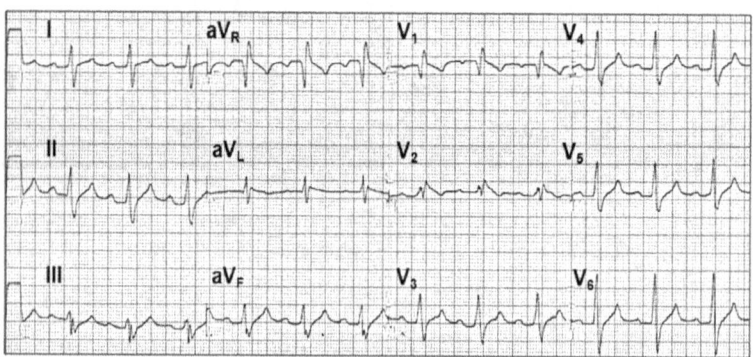

Chapter 11

Pediatric Electrocardiography

NORMAL PEDIATRIC ECG

The basic principles of cardiac conduction and depolarization are the same as for adults; however, features that would be diagnosed as abnormal in an adult's ECG may be normal in a pediatric ECG.

Pediatric Electrode Placement

Standard adult electrode positions are used. Leads V_3R and V_4R (and sometimes the extra posterior lead V_7) are occasionally used to provide additional information (Figure 11-1).

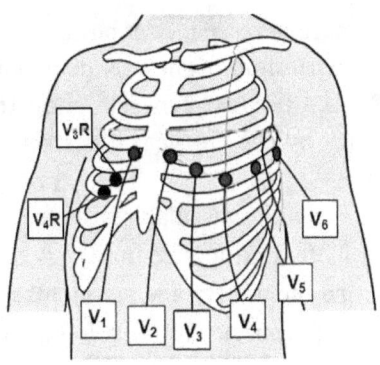

Figure 11-1. Pediatric electrode placement.

Heart Rate

In children, cardiac output is determined primarily by heart rate as opposed to stroke volume. With age, the heart rate decreases and stroke volume plays a larger role in determining cardiac output.

Age-appropriate heart rates must be taken into account when reading a pediatric ECG (Table 11-1). Heart rates significantly outside the normal range for age should be scrutinized for dysrhythmias.

Age	Heart rate (bpm)
1st wk	90–160
1–3 wk	100–180
1–2 mo	120–180
3–5 mo	105–185
6–11 mo	110–170
1–2 yr	90–165
3–4 yr	70–140
5–7 yr	65–140
8–11 yr	60–130
12–15 yr	65–130
>16 yr	50–120

Table 11-1. Heart rate as a function of age.

QRS Axis

Because of the high pulmonary vascular resistance at birth, the right ventricle is larger than the left. Therefore, right axis deviation is present. At birth, the mean QRS axis lies between +60° and +160°. The axis changes gradually so that by age one year it lies between +10° and +100° (Figures 11-2).

Changes in pulmonary and systemic vascular resistance with time result in the left ventricle increasing in size until it is larger than the right ventricle by age one month. By age six months, the ratio of the right ventricle to the left ventricle is similar to that of an adult.

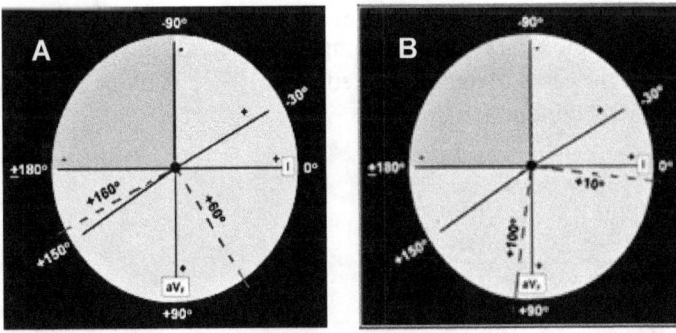

Figure 11-2. Axis: (A) birth and (B) One year.

PR Interval

The PR interval increases with age (Table 11-2). In neonates the PR interval ranges from 0.08–0.15 seconds and in adolescents from 0.12–0.20 seconds. The PR interval difference with age in children must be taken into account when considering the diagnosis of atrioventricular block.

Age	PR interval (seconds)
1st wk	0.08–0.15
1–3 wk	0.08–0.15
1–2 mo	0.08–0.15
3–5 mo	0.08–0.15
6–11 mo	0.07–0.16
1–2 yr	0.08–0.16
3–4 yr	0.09–0.17
5–7 yr	0.09–0.17
8–11 yr	0.09–0.17
12–15 yr	0.09–0.18
>16 yr	0.12–0.20

Table 11-2. PR interval as a function of age.

QRS Complex

In children, the QRS complex duration is shorter than in adults, and gradually increases with age. In neonates it is 0.03–0.08

seconds and in adolescents it is 0.05–0.10 seconds (Table 11-3). A QRS complex duration exceeding 0.08 seconds in children younger than eight years of age or exceeding 0.10 sec in older children may indicate a conduction delay.

Age	QRS interval (seconds)
1st wk	0.03–0.08
1–3 wk	0.03–0.08
1–2 mo	0.03–0.08
3–5 mo	0.03–0.08
6–11 mo	0.03–0.08
1–2 yr	0.03–0.08
3–4 yr	0.04–0.08
5–7 yr	0.04–0.08
8–11 yr	0.04–0.09
12–15 yr	0.04–0.09
>16 yr	0.05–0.10

Table 11-3. QRS interval as a function of age.

P Wave

The P wave is best evaluated from lead II, V_1, or V_{4R}. The normal height of the P wave is less than 3 mm in infants younger than six months of age and less than 2.5 mm in children older than six months of age. The P wave duration should be shorter than 0.12 seconds.

T waves

Flat or inverted T waves are normal in the newborn. T waves in leads V_1-V_3 usually are inverted after the first week of life through the age of eight years. However, this pattern can persist into early adolescence.

QT Interval

Because the QT interval varies greatly with heart rate as in adults, it is usually corrected to QTc.

During the first half of infancy, the normal QTc is longer than in older children and adults. In the first six months of life, QTc is considered normal if it is less than 0.49 seconds. After infancy, the cut-off is 0.44 seconds in males and 0.46 seconds in males.

Other ECG Findings in Infants and Young Children

Dominant right precordial R waves in leads V_1-V_3 are normal. Inferior and lateral Q waves in leads II, III, aV_F, and V_6 are also normal. An RSR' may be present in lead V_1

Summary of Pediatric ECG Findings that May Be Normal

* Heart rate > 100 bpm
* QRS axis > +90° (RAD)
* Right precordial T wave inversion (leads V_1-V_3)
* Dominant right precordial R waves (leads V_1-V_3)
* Short PR and long QT intervals
* Short duration of QRS complexes
* Inferior and lateral Q waves in leads II, III, aV_F, and V_6.
* P wave amplitude varies little with age after six months of age.
* You may see an RSR' in lead V_1.

A normal pediatric ECG is shown in Figure 11-3.

ABNORMAL PEDIATRIC ECG

Chamber Size

Chamber size refers to right and left ventricular hypertrophy and right and left atrial enlargement.

Right Ventricular Hypertrophy Criteria

* R wave greater than the upper limit of normal in lead V_1
* S wave greater than the upper limit of normal in lead

I or lead V₆

- RSR' pattern in lead V_1, with the R' height being greater than 1.5 mV in infants younger than 1 year of age or greater than 1.0 mV in children older than 1 year of age
- Q wave in lead V_1

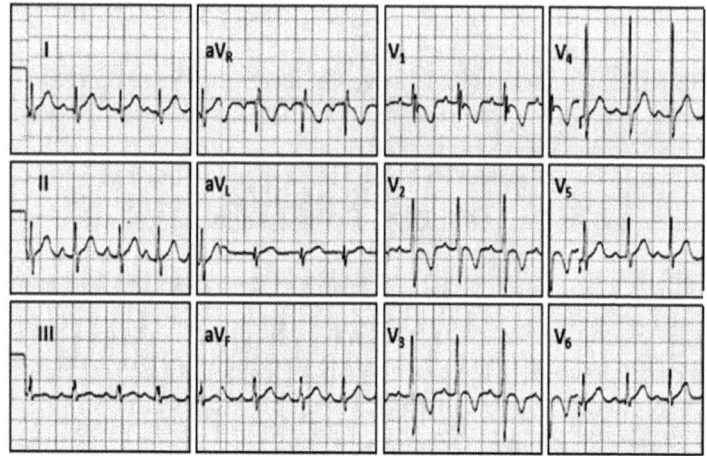

Figure 11-3. Normal ECG for a two-year old child. Note a heart rate of greater than 100 bpm, dominant R waves in leads V_1-V_3, RSR' in lead V_1, and T wave inversion in leads V_1- V_3.

Table 11-4 shows R and S waves in various leads as a function of age.

Age	R in V₁ (mm)	S in V₁ (mm)	R in V₆ (mm)	S in V₆ (mm)
1st wk	5–26	0–23	0–12	0–10
1–3 wk	3–21	0–16	2–16	0–10
1–2 mo	3–18	0–15	5–21	0–10
3–5 mo	3–20	0–15	6–22	0–10
6–11 mo	2–20	0.5–20	6–23	0–7
1–2 yr	2–18	0.5–21	6–23	0–7
3–4 yr	1–18	0.5–21	4–24	0–5
5–7 yr	0.5–14	0.5–24	4–26	0–4
8–11 yr	0–14	0.5–25	4–25	0–4
12–15 yr	0–14	0.5–21	4–25	0–4
>16 yr	0–14	0.5–23	4–21	0–4

Table 11-4. R and S waves in various leads as a function of age.

Left Ventricular Hypertrophy Criteria

- R-wave amplitude greater than upper limit of normal in lead V_5 or V_6
- R wave less than the lower limit of normal in lead V_1 or V_2
- S-wave amplitude greater than the upper limit of normal in lead V_1
- Q wave greater than 4 mm in lead V_5 or V_6
- Inverted T wave in lead V_6

Biventricular hypertrophy

- ECG criteria for enlargement of both ventricles

Right Atrial Enlargement Criteria

- Peaked P waves in leads II and V_1 that are higher than 3 mm in infants younger than six months of age and greater than 2.5 mm in infants older than six months of age

Left Atrial Enlargement Criteria

- P-wave duration greater than 0.08 seconds in children younger than 12 months of age or greater than 10 ms in children one year and older
- Terminal or deeply inverted P wave in lead V_1 or V_{3R}

AV Block

All degrees of AV block may occur in pediatric patients. The normal PR interval in infants is shorter than in adults and lengthens as the child gets older.

A PR interval approaching 0.20 seconds, which is normal in an adult, may represent a first-degree AV block in an infant or young child.

Bundle branch blocks may be present when there is QRS complex prolongation abnormal for a given age. Right bundle branch block occurs with abnormal rightward forces. It is frequently manifesting on an ECG as an RSR' pattern in leads V_1 and V_2, although this may be normal in young children.

Left BBB bundle branch block is seen with abnormal leftward forces, best appreciated in leads V_5 and V_6. Left bundle branch block is rare in children; however, the possibility of Wolff-Parkinson-White syndrome should be considered because this syndrome can mimic a left bundle branch block.

Tachydysrhythmias

As in adults, tachydysrhythmias can be classified as supraventricular (arise above the AV node), AV node reentry tachycardias (originate from the AV node), and ventricular (arise in the ventricles).

The vast majority of tachycardias in children are supraventricular in origin, with sinus tachycardia being the most common. The peak incidence of supraventricular tachycardia occurs during the first two months of life.

Infants with supraventricular tachycardia have fussiness, poor feeding, pallor, or lethargy; whereas older children complain of chest pain, pounding in the chest, dizziness, or shortness of breath.

In newborns and young infants, pulse rate with supraventricular tachycardia can be 250 to 300 beats per minute. In older children it is usually less than 250 bpm and may be in the range of 180 to 200 bpm in teenagers.

The normal QRS complex is shorter in duration in children than adults; as a result, a tachycardia with a QRS complex width of 0.09 seconds, which is normal for an adult, represents an abnormally wide QRS complex tachycardia in an infant.

Indications for a Pediatric ECG

Chest pain in children is rarely cardiac in origin and is often associated with tenderness in the chest wall. Indications for pediatric electrocardiography are given in Table 11-5.

Table 11-5. Indications for pediatric electrocardiology.

• Syncope or seizure	• Electrolyte disturbance
• Exertional symptoms	• Kawasaki disease
• Drug ingestion	• Rheumatic fever
• Tachyarrhythmia	• Myocarditis
• Bradyarrhythmia	• Myocardial contusion
• Cyanotic episodes	• Pericarditis
• Heart failure	• Post cardiac surgery
• Hypothermia	• Congenital heart defects

Congenital Heart Defects

Infants with congenital heart defects may present with tachypnea and sudden onset of cyanosis or pallor, lethargy, or failure to thrive. Symptoms may worsen with crying, sweating, or feeding. Table 11-6 gives the classification of common congenital heart defects.

Table 11-6. Classification of congenital heart defects.

Acyanotic	Cyanotic
• **Obstructive Lesions**	• **Right-to-left shunt lesions**
• Pulmonary stenosis	• Tetralogy of Fallot
• Aortic stenosis	• Transposition of the great arteries
• Coarctation of the aorta	• Tricuspid atresia
• **Left-to-right shunt lesions**	
• Atrial septal defect	
• Ventricular septal defect	
• Patent ductus arteriosus	

First Two to Three Weeks of Life

Congenital heart disease that presents in the first two to three weeks of life is typically the result of closure of the ductus arteriosus, which had been sustaining blood flow. This occurs with tetralogy of Fallot, tricuspid atresia, coarctation of the aorta, and hypoplastic left heart syndrome. When the ductus closes, these infants suddenly develop symptoms of cyanosis or signs of cardiovascular collapse.

Other Defects that Present in the First Month

The other class of congenital cardiac defects that present in the first month of life are the left-to-right intracardiac shunts, such as:

- Ventricular septal
- Atrioventricular canal defects.

Over the first month of life, as the normal pulmonary vascular resistance falls, a gradual increase in flow across a pre-existing left-to-right shunt takes place, resulting in congestive heart failure.

Common ECG Findings with Congenital Heart Defects

Some common ECG findings that may appear with congenital heart defects include:

Axis Deviation

- **Right axis deviation** can occur with atrial septal defect, tetralogy of Fallot, coarctation of the aorta, transposition of the great arteries, and pulmonary stenosis.

- **Left axis deviation** can be seen with large ventricular septal defect, tricuspid atresia, transposition of the great arteries, and complete AV canal defects.

Bundle Branch Blocks

- **Right bundle branch block** can be seen with atrial septal defect, complete AV defects, and small ventricular septal defects.

- **Left bundle branch block,** as mentioned before, is rare in children; however, the possibility of Wolff-Parkinson-White syndrome should be considered because this syndrome can mimic a left bundle branch block.

Ventricular Hypertrophy

- **Right ventricular hypertrophy** is the most common abnormality seen with congenital heart disease. It can be seen with pulmonary stenosis, tetralogy of Fallot, transposition of the great arteries, and ventricular septal defect, pulmonary stenosis, and pulmonary hypertension, coarctation of the aorta, pulmonary valve atresia, hypoplastic left heart syndrome, and atrial septal   defect.

  Right ventricle hypertrophy may be difficult to assess during the early neonatal period because of the normal right ventricular predominance at this age. The abnormality becomes clear, however, as the child becomes older.

- **Left ventricular hypertrophy** is seen in lesions with small right ventricles, such as tricuspid atresia, pulmonary atresia with an intact ventricular septum, and lesions with left ventricular outflow track obstruction, such as aortic stenosis, coarctation of the aorta, and hypertrophic cardiomyopathy. Left ventricular hypertrophy also can be seen in older children with patent ductus arteriosis and large ventricular septal defect and atrioventricular canal defects.

Atrial Enlargement

- **Right atrial enlargement** occurs with large left-to-right shunts, causing right atrium volume overload, and can be seen with ASD, atrioventricular canal defects, tricuspid atresia, Ebstein anomaly, and severe pulmonary stenosis.
- **Left atrial enlargement** can be seen with mitral stenosis, mitral insufficiency, left heart outflow obstruction, and atrioventricular canal defects.

An ECG should be obtained in all infants suspected of having congenital heart disease. Although the ECG does not make the diagnosis, it can show evidence of abnormalities associated with congenital heart defects. These infants should be referred promptly, preferably to a pediatric cardiologist if one is available.

Chapter 11 Quiz

1. The normal axis of newborns is normally
   A. Normal axis
   B. Left axis
   C. Right axis
   D. Gray zone
   E. Norwest axis

2. The PR interval in young children
   A. Decreases with age
   B. Increases with age
   C. Does not change with age
   D. Does not depend on age
   E. Both increases and decreases with age (Schrodinger's PR interval)

3. T waves in leads V_1-V_3 in young children between one week and 8 years of age are usually _____
   A. Tall and peaked
   B. Very wide
   C. Very Narrow
   D. Inverted
   E. Nonexistent

4. In young children you may see an RR' in lead
   A. I
   B. III

C. V$_1$

D. V$_3$

E. V$_6$

5. In children, cardiac output is determined primarily by heart rate or stroke volume?

6. By age _____ the ratio of the right ventricle to the left ventricle is similar to that of an adult.
   A. 3 months
   B. 6 months
   C. 9 months
   D. 12 months

7. In the first 6 months of life, QTc is considered abnormal if it is greater than _____ seconds.
   A. 0.41 seconds
   B. 0.43 seconds
   C. 0.46 seconds
   D. 0. 49 seconds

8. The vast majority of tachycardias in children are _____.
   A. Atrial fibrillation
   B. Sinus tachycardia
   C. Multifocal
   D. Atrial flutter

9. The most common abnormality seen with congenital heart disease is _____.

   A. Right ventricular hypertrophy
   B. Left ventricular hypertrophy
   C. Left atrial enlargement
   D. Right atrial enlargement

Appendix A

ECG Findings for Specific Congenital Heart Defects

Acyanotic defects

Obstructive lesions.

- **Pulmonary stenosis.** The ECG shows right ventricular hypertrophy, the degree of which is proportional to the severity of the stenosis. Right atrial enlargement may be present.

- **Aortic stenosis.** The ECG may be normal or may show varying degrees of left ventricular hypertrophy. Inverted T waves in the left chest leads indicate that aortic valve obstruction is severe. However, not all severe AS patients show T wave inversion.

- **Coarctation of the aorta.** The ECG may be normal or may show left ventricular hypertrophy.

Left-to-right shunt lesions

- **Atrial septal defect.** The ECG shows mild right ventricular hypertrophy, and my show the diastolic volume overload pattern with RSR' pattern in the right chest leads.

- **Ventricular septal defect.** The ECG may be normal in very small defects or may show evidence for left ventricular hypertrophy in small to moderate defects while it may show biventricular or right ventricular hypertrophy in large defects. Electrocardiographic signs of left atrial enlargement may also be seen.

- **Patent ductus arteriosus.** The ECG may be normal or may show left atrial and left ventricular enlargement, depending upon the size of the ductus.

Cyanotic defects

Right-to-left shunts

- **Tetralogy of Fallot.** The ECG shows signs of right ventricular hypertrophy. Right atrial enlargement is less commonly seen.

- **Transposition of the great vessels.** Group I: The ECG in a neonate with transposition of the great vessels and intact septum may be normal with the usual right ventricular preponderance seen in neonates. In older infants clear-cut right ventricular hypertrophy is seen and in addition right atrial enlargement may be observed.

  - Group II: Biventricular hypertrophy and left atrial enlargement are usually seen.

  - Group III: Right ventricular or biventricular enlargement is seen.

- **Tricuspid atresia.** The ECG can be virtually diagnostic of tricuspid atresia in an infant with cyanotic congestive heart failure. The characteristic features include:

  - Right atrial enlargement
  - Left axis deviation
  - Left ventricular hypertrophy
  - Diminished right ventricular forces.

Appendix B
Practice ECGs

Interpret the following ECGs. Use the 8-step form given in Chapter 10.

1.

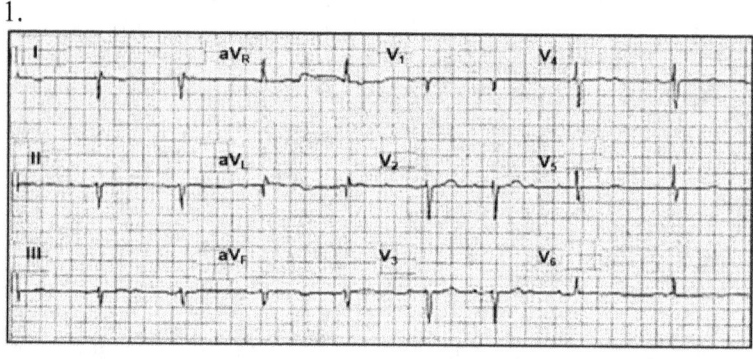

2.

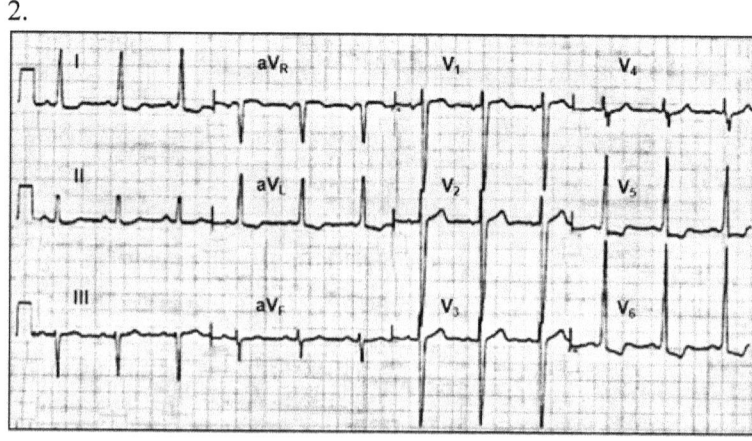

3.

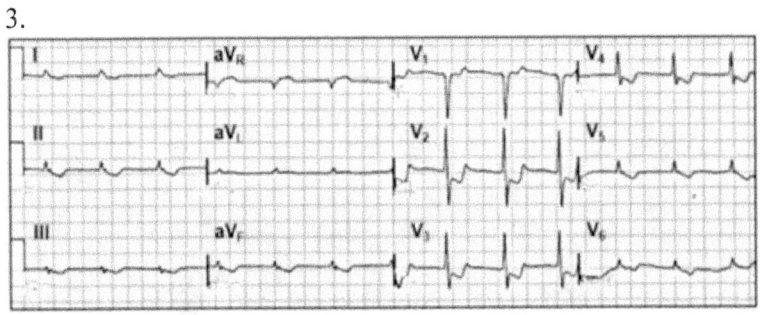

4.

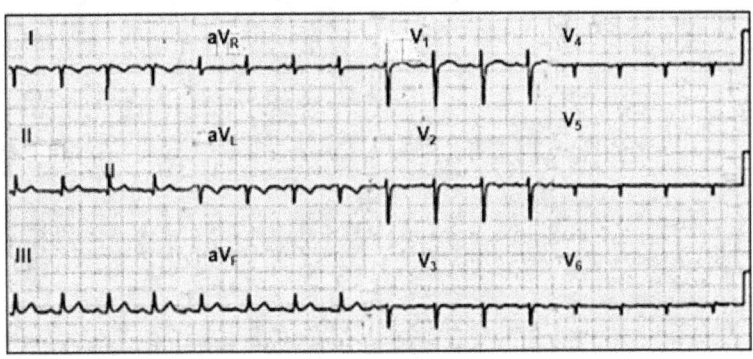

5.

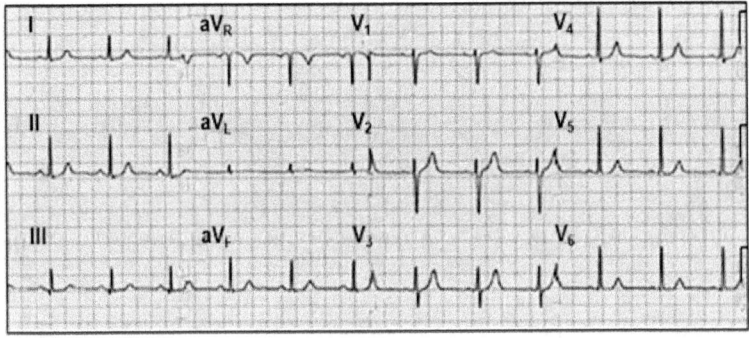

6.

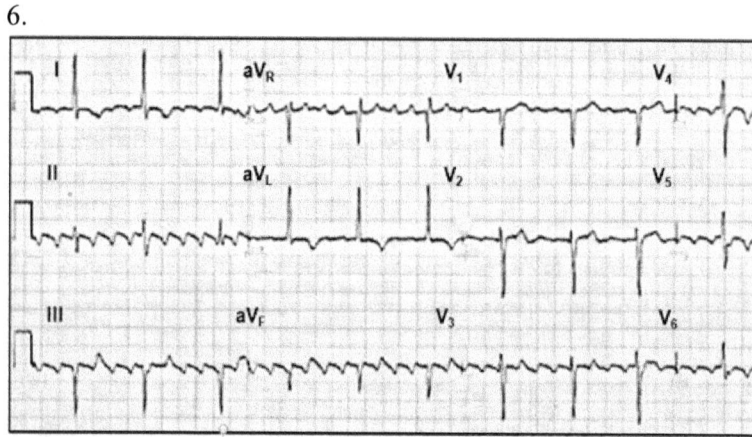

7.

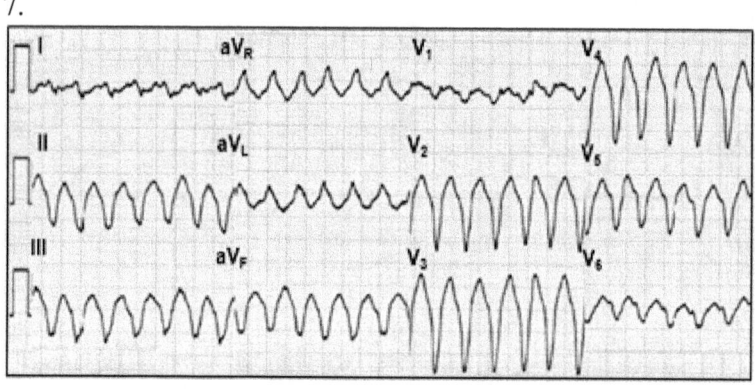

8.

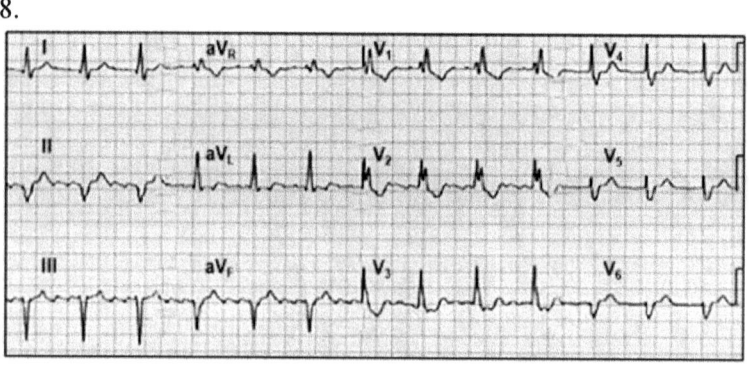

9.

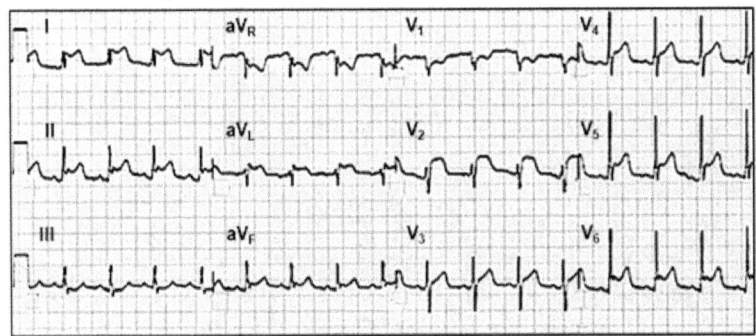

10.

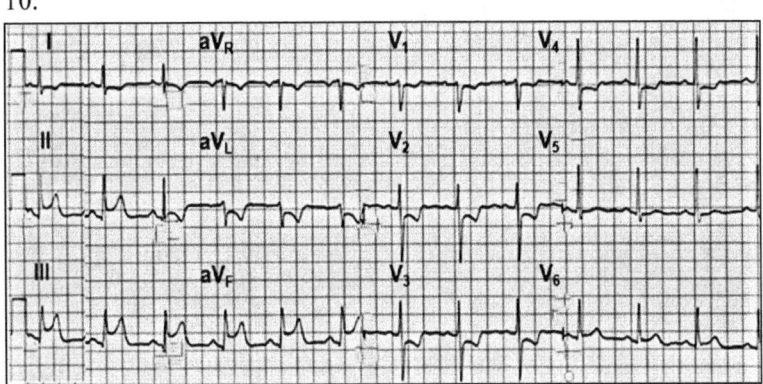

11.

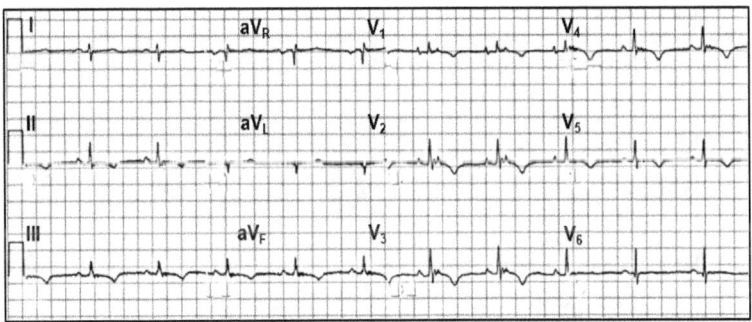

Appendix C

Answers to Chapter Questions and Practice ECGs

Chapter 1
1. 0.5 mV
2. 0.2 seconds
3. 0.04 seconds
4. 0.1 mV
5. E
6. D
7. A
8. B
9. C
10. 0.4
11. F
12. D
13. B
14. E
15. C
16. A
17. G
18. 0.545
19. Prolonged

Chapter 2

1. 0.48
2. 0.48
3. Prolonged
4. Normal
5.

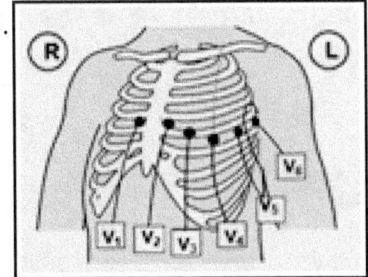

6. Bipolar

7. Unipolar

8. Unipolar

9. I

10. III

11. II

12. I, aV_L, V_5, V_6

13. II, III, aV_F

14. V_3, V_4

15. V_1, V_2

16. D

Chapter 3

1. 100 bpm
2. 50 bpm
3. 30 bpm
4. QT – 0.280 seconds
5. QTc = 0.438 seconds
6. LAD zone
7. Normal range, normal zone
8. Northwest axis zone
9. RAD zone

    10. Normal range, Gray zone

Chapter 4
   1. 2.5 mm
   2. 0.11 seconds
   3. T
   4. F
   5. T
   6. Biatrial enlargement
   7. Right atrial enlargement
   8. Left atrial enlargement
   9. Biventricular hypertrophy
   10. Left ventricular hypertrophy
   11. Right ventricular hypertrophy

Chapter 5
   1. Septum
   2. Left bundle branch
   3. Right
   4. Left
   5. RBBB
   6. LBBB
   7. LAD
   8. RAD
   9. False
   10. RBBB
   11. LBBB
   12. Left anterior hemiblock
   13. Left posterior hemiblock

Chapter 6
   1. D
   2. F
   3. B
   4. C
   5. A
   6. C
   7. A
   8. B

9. Posterior STEMI
10. Anterior STEMI
11. Inferior STEMI
12. LV aneurysm
13. Old inferior STEMI
14. Inferior STEMI with right ventricular infarct
15. Wellen's syndrome

Chapter 7
1. Electrical alternans
2. Supraventricular tachycardia
3. Sick sinus syndrome
4. Ventricular tachycardia
5. Sinus bradycardia
6. Premature atrial contraction
7. Bigeminy
8. Junctional rhythm
9. Junctional escape beat
10. Torsades de pointes
11. Multifocal atrial tachycardia
12. Atrial flutter
13. 2nd degree block, Mobitz type I
14. Premature junctional beat
15. Normal sinus rhythm
16. Atrial fibrillation
17. PVC
18. Ventricular fibrillation
19. First degree heart block
20. Ventricular tachycardia
21. Supraventricular Beat with aberrancy
22. Third degree heart block

Chapter 8
1. F
2. Clockwise
3. WPW with AF
4. T
5. A
6. B
7. WPW

8. Pericarditis
9. Early repolarization
10. LGL
11. Myocarditis
12. Pulmonary embolus ($S_1Q_3T_3$)

Chapter 9
1. B
2. D
3. C
4. F
5. Normal
6. Brugada syndrome, type 2
7. Low-voltage
8. Hypothermia
9. Brugada syndrome, type 1
10. Neurological insult
11. Dextrocardia

Chapter 10
1. C
2. C
3. A
4. C
5. Short
6. Hyperkalemia, severe
7. Hypocalcemia
8. Digoxin toxicity
9. Digoxin effect
10. Hyperkalemia, moderate
11. TCA overdose

Chapter 11
1. C
2. B
3. D
4. C
5. Heart rate
6. B
7. D

8. B
9. A

Answers for practice ECGs in Appendix B
1. bradycardia, Northwest axis
2. LVH with strain
3. Posterior MI
4. Situs inversus
5. normal
6. Atrial flutter
7. Ventricular tachycardia
8. RBBB
9. Pericarditis
10. Inferior STEMI
11. Arrhythmogenic right ventricular dysplasia

References

1. Argyle, Bruce, MicroEKG, http://www.madsci.com/manu/in-dexekg.htm.
2. Blake, T. M. Introduction to Electrocardiography. Appleton-Century Crofts, New York, 1972.
3. Braunwald's Heart Disease: A Textbook of Cardiovascular Medicine, 10th edition. Edited by Douglas L. Mann et al. Elsevier, Philadelphia, 2015.
4. Burns, Edward, Life in the Fastlane, http://lifeinthefastlane.com/ecg-library/basics/\
5. Chang, Henry, James K. Min, Sunil V. Rao, Manesh R. Patel, Orlando P. Simonetti, Giuseppe Ambrosio, and Subha V. Raman. Non–ST-Segment Elevation Acute Coronary Syndromes Targeted Imaging to Refine Upstream Risk Stratification, Circulation: Cardiovascular Imaging. 2012;5:536-546.
6. Chapter 8: Cardiology and Vascular Disease, TheDoctorsLounge.net, http://www.thedoctorslounge.net/ linlounge/diseases/cardiology/.
7. De Jong, Jonas, www.ECGpedia.org.
8. Drugs which cause QT interval prolongation, DrugIntel Newsletter, http://www.drugintel.com/drugs/qt_arrhythmia.htm, February 14, 2003.
9. Dubin, D. Rapid Interpretation of EKG's, 6th edition. Cover Publishing Col, Tampa, 2000.
10. ECG Library, Contents, http://www.ecglibrary.com/ecghome.html.
11. EKG, FamilyPracticeNotebook.com, http://www.fpnotebook.com/CV52.htm.
12. EKG of the week, http://jhcedecg.blogspot.com/p/ecg-reference-notes.html
13. Electrocardiogram in Pericarditis, FamilyPracticeNote-

book.com, http://www.fpnotebook.com/CV76.htm.

14. Electrocardiograms, Interpretation of (Position Paper), Policy & Advocacy, AAFP, http://www.aafp.org/x6765.xml.

15. Electrocardiography, Echo services, http://www.echo-services.com.au/EchoSpeak/FAQ/Electrocardiography.aspx, 2002.

16. Electrocardiography, Health Guide A - Z, WebMD, http://my.webmd.com/hw/heart_disease/hw213248.asp.

17. Electrocardiography: An Overview, Catcha.com.My, http://www.catcha.com.my/channels/health/content_page.pht ml?main=cardiology20.my.

18. Froom, J. and P. T. Tchao. A Curriculum in Electrocardiography for Family Physicians, J. Fam. Pract. 5:857-863, 1981.

19. Goldberger, A. L. and E. Goldberger. Clinical Electrocardiography, C. V. Mosby Co., St. Louis, 2012.

20. Goodacre, Steve and Karen McLeod, *ABC of clinical electrocardiography,* Paediatric electrocardiography, BMJ VOLUME 324 8 June 2002.

21. Gottlieb, S. H. D. D. Zieve, and G. C. Voight. Arrhythmias, In Principles of Ambulatory Medicine, 7th edition. Ed. by L. R. Barker, J. R. Burton, and J. R. Zieve. Williams and Wilkins Co., 2006.

22. Grauer, Ken, 12-lead ECGs: A Pocket Brain for Easy Interpretation (6th Edition), Kg/EKG Press, Gainesville, 2013.

23. Haddad, A. and D. C. Dean. Interpreting EKGs. Medical Economics Co. Oradell, New Jersey, 1981.

24. Hals, Gary D. and Stephen C. Carleton, Pericardial Disease, http://www.hypertension-consult.com/Secure/textbook articles/Textbook/59_pericardial.htm.

25. Hodges M, Salerno D, Erlien D. *(*1983*)* Bazett's QT correction reviewed-evidence that a linear QT correction for heart is better. *J Am Coll Cardiol* 1*:*694.

26. Iqbal, Itif, EKG Case #2 – Acute Pericarditis, Albany Medical Review, http://www.amc.edu/amr/archives/200408/ekg2_ans.html, August 2004.

27. Jenkins, Dean and Stephen Gerred. ECG Library, Contents, http://www.ecglibrary.com/.

28. Lome, Steven D.O., LearnTheHeart, http://www.learntheheart.com

29. Marinella, Mark A, Electrocardiographic Manifestations and

Differential Diagnosis of Acute Pericarditis, AFP, Feb 15;57(4):699-704, 1998.

30. Martin, Gary and Arnold S. Baas, S-T-Elevation/Q-Wave Myocardial Infarction, Best Practice of Medicine, January 2004.
31. Meter, M. V. and P. G. Lavine. Reading EKGs Correctly, 2nd edition. Nursing 77 Books Springhouse Publishing Co, 1984.
32. Milhorn, H. T. Jr. Electrocardiography for the Family Physician: Part I. Family Practice Recertification, 5(2)69-94, 1983.
33. Milhorn, H. T. Jr. Electrocardiography for the Family Physician: Part II. Family Practice Recertification, 5(3)105-130, 1983.
34. Milhorn, H. T. Jr. Electrocardiography for the Family Physician: Part III. Family Practice Recertification, 5(4)35-57, 1983.
35. Milhorn, H. T. Jr. Electrocardiography for the Family Physician: Part IV. Family Practice Recertification, 5(5)101-124, 1983.
36. Milhorn, H. T. Jr. Electrocardiography for the Family Physician: Part V. Family Practice Recertification, 5(6)121-137, 1983.
37. Mudge, G. H. Manual of Electrocardiography, 2nd edition. Little-Brown and Co., Boston, 1981
38. Outline of interactive electrocardiography, EKG Section, Loyola University Chicago, Stritch School of Medicine, http://www.meddean.luc.edu/lumen/MedEd/MEDICINE/medc lerk/ekg.htm.
39. Rao, P. Syamasundar, University of Texas at Houston Medical School, Houston, http://cdn.intechweb.org/pdfs/26653.pdf.
40. Sgarbossa, E., et al. (1996). Electrocardiographic diagnosis of evolving acute myocardial infarction in the presence of left bundle-branch block. The New England Journal of Medicine. *334*, 481-487.
41. Sharieff, Ghazala Q. and Sri O. Rao The Pediatric ECG, Emerg Med Clin N Am 24 (2006) 195–208.
42. Takotsubo cardiomyopathy, WikiEcho, http://www.wikiecho .org /wiki/Takotsubo_cardiomyopathy
43. Tempelhof, Michael W, EKG an overview and tutorial for residents teaching medical students, http://www.askdrwiki .com/mediawiki/index.php?title=EKG_an_overview_and_tutorial_for_residents_teaching_medical_students

44. Torsade de Pointe, eMedicine.com, http://www.cmcdi-cine.com/MED/topic2286ıhtm#section~wor kup, 2005.
45. Wagner, Galen S. and David D. Strauss, Marriott's Practical Electrocardiography, 12th edition, Lippincott Williams & Wilkins, 2013.
46. Yanowitz, Frank, **G.**, ECG Learning Center, An introduction to clinical electrocardiography, http://ecg.utah.edu/outline.

Acknowledgements

- Table 8-1 is based on Iqbal, Itif, EKG Case #2 – Acute Pericard-tis, Albany Medical Review, http://www.amc.edu/amr/archives/ 200408/EKG2_ans.html, August 2004.
- Tables 11-1 to 11-4 and the criteria for abnormal ECGs are based on Sharieff, Ghazala Q. and Sri O. Rao The Pediatric ECG, Emerg Med Clin N Am 24 (2006) 195–208
- Table 11-5 and Figure 11-3 are based on Goodacre, Steve and Karen McLeod, *ABC of clinical electrocardiography,* Paediatric electrocardiography, BMJ Volume 324 8 June 2002.
- Table 11-6 and the discussion of ECG findings in congenital heart disease are based on Rao, P. Syamasundar, University of Texas at Houston Medical School, Houston, ttp://cdn.inte-chweb.org/ pdfs/26653.pdf.

Index

Other Books by H. Thomas Milhorn

1. Substance Use Disorders: A Guide for the Primary Care Provider, Springer, 2017.
2. Electrocardiography for the Family Physician: The Essentials, Second Edition, Universal Publishers, 2014.
3. The History of Physics, Virtual Bookworm, 2008.
4. The History of Astronomy and Astrophysics, Virtual Bookworm, 2008.
5. Cybercrime: How to Avoid Becoming a Victim, Universal Publishers, 2007.
6. Writing Genre Fiction: A Guide to the Craft, Universal Publishers 2006.
7. Crime: Computer Viruses to Twin Towers, Universal Publishers, 2005.
8. Drug and Alcohol Abuse: The Authoritative Guide for Parents, Teachers and Counselors, Da Capo, 2003.
9. Caduceus Awry (a medical thriller), Writer's Showcase, 2000.
10. Chemical Dependence: Diagnosis, Treatment, and Prevention, Springer-Verlag, 1990.
11. The Application of Control Theory to Physiological Systems, W. B. Saunders, 1966.